英汉对比语言学研究丛书

英汉疾病隐喻的认知对比研究

Cognitive and Contrastive Analysis of Disease Metaphors in English and Chinese

刘 晓 著

本书获江苏省哲学社会科学重大项目(2020SJZDA013)、教育部人文社科青年基金项目(22YJC740049)资助。

苏州大学出版社

图书在版编目(CIP)数据

英汉疾病隐喻的认知对比研究 = Cognitive and Contrastive Analysis of Disease Metaphors in English and Chinese：英文／刘晓著. --苏州：苏州大学出版社，2024.8. --(英汉对比语言学研究丛书).
ISBN 978-7-5672-4755-0

Ⅰ．R441；H314

中国国家版本馆 CIP 数据核字第 202469MA37 号

英汉疾病隐喻的认知对比研究

书　　名：	Cognitive and Contrastive Analysis of Disease Metaphors in English and Chinese
著　者：	刘　晓
责任编辑：	汤定军
策划编辑：	汤定军
封面设计：	刘　俊
出版发行：	苏州大学出版社(Soochow University Press)
社　　址：	苏州市十梓街 1 号　邮编：215006
印　　装：	江苏凤凰数码印务有限公司
网　　址：	www.sudapress.com
邮　　箱：	sdcbs@suda.edu.cn
邮购热线：	0512-67480030
销售热线：	0512-67481020
开　　本：	700 mm×1 000 mm　1/16　印张：12.75　字数：229 千
版　　次：	2024 年 8 月第 1 版
印　　次：	2024 年 8 月第 1 次印刷
书　　号：	ISBN 978-7-5672-4755-0
定　　价：	58.00 元

凡购本社图书发现印装错误，请与本社联系调换。服务热线：0512-67481020

Contents

Introduction / 1

Chapter 1 Metaphor as a Lens to Mind / 8
    1.1 Metaphor as a Way of Cognition / 10
    1.2 Metaphor's Role in Lexical Meaning Extension / 16
    1.3 Cross-Cultural Cognitive Studies through Metaphors / 21
    1.4 Bibliometric Analysis of Studies on Disease Metaphors / 24

Chapter 2 Corpus-Based Comparison of Disease Metaphors in English and Chinese / 29
    2.1 Corpus-Based Comparison of Semantic Themes of Disease Metaphors in English and Chinese / 30
    2.2 Distribution of Typical Conceptual Metaphors in the Self-Established Corpus of *China Daily* and BBC News / 57
    2.3 Further Analysis of Contradictory Themes from Two Sources / 84
    2.4 Visualization of Key Metaphor Words in *China Daily* and BBC News / 92

Chapter 3 Spatial-Temporal Cognition Analysis of Disease Metaphors in English and Chinese / 108
    3.1 Different Disease Metaphors with "Root" in English and 根 in Chinese / 109
    3.2 Corpus-Based Analysis of Disease Metaphors with Chinese 根 and English "Root" / 116
    3.3 Spatial-Temporal Cognition of the Word Meaning Construal Between 根 and "Root" / 123

Chapter 4 Similarities and Differences in the Schematization of Disease and 疾 / 129
    4.1 Space-Oriented Cognition in Chinese vs Time-Oriented Cognition in English / 131
    4.2 Comparison of the Image Schemas of Frequent Disease Metaphors with 根/Root / 136

4.3　Differences in Schematization of the Disease Metaphor with 根 and "Root"　／140

4.4　Sign Language Evidence for Different Perspectives in Viewing 根 and "Root"　／147

Chapter 5　Social-Cultural Analysis of Differences in Expressing Causes of Diseases in English and Chinese　／150

5.1　Differences in Expressions for Causative Motions Between English and Chinese　／152

5.2　Social-Cultural Factors for Different Semantic Restraints for Causative Motions　／157

5.3　Force Dynamic Analysis of Causative Motions　／165

5.4　Summary of the Analysis of Causation and Its Implication in Understanding Causes for Disease in English and Chinese　／177

References　／189

Introduction

Mental process represents the experiential meaning of the inner world in the transitivity system. In other words, it describes the occurrence and development of people's psychological activities, and reflects human brain to reality. Mental process can be divided into four types: emotive process, desiderative process, perceptive process and cognitive process. Despite the various emphases on what goes on inside human mind, all the above processes have three things in common, that is, all of them require sensor, phenomenon, and can be reflected in the language used by the sensor.

As one of the oldest universal phenomena, illness is frequently talked about in different languages and cultures. The author of this book believes that the words, phrases, and conventionalized syntax used in discussing illness or disease in different languages have substantial influence on how the native speakers of that language community feel, perceive, and understand illness. The argument about the relationship between language and the worldview of its users can date back to the famous German linguist Humbolt in the 19th century, who has pioneered the hypothesis between language and its influence on worldview in the publication of *The Heterogeneity of Language and Its Influence on the Intellectual Development of Mankind*. Humbolt is often referred to as the originator of the later Sapir-Whorf hypothesis in the early 20th century, suggesting that the structure of a language influences its speakers' worldview or cognition, and thus people's perceptions are relative to their spoken language. The hypothesis is also known as linguistic relativity. There have been stronger and weaker versions of linguistic relativity, of which the stronger version is now referred to as linguistic determinism, saying that a language determines thought and that linguistic categories limit and determine cognitive categories. The stronger version of linguistic relativity has gradually been deserted in modern linguistics. The study concerning the relationship between language and mind continued to develop. Humbolt (1999) discussed how language can influence and be influenced by national character and spirit. Cognitive linguists also upheld that the ability to use language taps into the same reservoir that ensures the development of cognitive competence (Lakoff & Johnson, 2008; Langacker, 1987; Talmy, 2000). The position of this book adopts the middle line, which is more consistent with Hombolt and general cognitive linguistics, arguing that the language used by people in discussing illness will not "shape" their cognition, but definitely cast a strong shadow. Furthermore, the emotion, attitude, and cognition revealed in the language employed in discussing illness can affect how they respond to the illness and disease in the real world, as well as how they tend to treat the illness and handle the disease. Therefore, by analyzing the languages used to talk about illness, we can gain a deeper understanding about why people from different language communities and cultures may have different responses to the same disease. Here the responses include both emotional and perceptual differences. Moreover, an enhanced mutual understanding can minimize the possibility of misunderstanding across cultures and curb the spread of misinformation. Considering the international disputes over corona virus in the past three years and the measures to prevent the pandemic, effective cultural exchanges and communication become both necessary and urgent. For the lack of deepened mutual understanding can be easily twisted, distorted, and spread very quickly in today's media, explanation and countermeasures can only ease the negative influence to a limited degree. The fundamental long-term approach in dealing with the spread of misinformation is through enhanced cultural exchanges, that's because misinformation has to be built on the lack of knowledge and inherent stereotype. So if we can present the real image of a country with profound knowledge and cultural backgrounds, the biased stereotype that feeds on ambiguity and hearsay will gradually disappear. And when there is no public foundation for the spread of misinformation, the fake news and biased interpretation will naturally die out.

  Now that the significance of analyzing the language used to talk about illness is proven, what is left is to further clarify what kind of language is more worthy of our attention. The assumption we adopt here is that the more conventionalized the expression is, the more likely it can reflect the fixed cognitive pattern of the speakers. Here the more conventionalized expression enjoys three features: first, it has a rather fixed and rigid form for its users to apply; second, it is developed based on universal cognitive principles of human beings; third, it is rooted in the daily practice of the users. These three features can guarantee both the feasibility and the value of the study. For the discussion of all linguistic expressions used to discuss illness is both impossible and pointless, paying attention to fixed phraseology is a more plausible option. Besides, the so-called "fixed" expressions become fossilized due to their frequent usage and wide adoption among the language users in the community, thus making them a suitable object to study common emotion, perception and cognition. Moreover, the expressions are rooted in daily practice, which makes them a possible reflection of people's value and worldview in reality. Considering the above three features, one of the most suitable phraseology we can use as a lens to investigate the language users' perception and cognition of illness or disease is metaphor. Metaphor is a conventionalized expression abstracted from common daily practice, which is featured by the relatively fixed language form. Besides, given that the living environment of human beings has many similarities, there are certain conceptual metaphors, such as space, time, and journey, which are prevalent among different languages and cultures, providing the precondition for cross-cultural analysis.

The existing studies of disease metaphors usually pay more attention to the evident and novel metaphors, that is, metaphors with a higher degree of metaphoricity. Apart from the in-balanced distribution between novel metaphors and "dead" metaphors, there is also a lack of cross-language comparison between disease metaphors, especially diachronic comparison that analyzes the meaning extension of words or phrases used to denote illness. Besides, the methods used in analyzing disease metaphors are limited to case analysis based on linguistic theories, and corpus-based metaphor study is still insufficient. Furthermore, the study of word semantics is separated into the traditional word meaning study, which is classified as lexicography, and cognitive semantics, which focuses on the cognitive reasons for the word meaning extension. However, the problem is there is no clear demarcation between the original basic word meaning study and its meaning extension. The traditional lexicography also needs to consider people's cognition of words, and the relatively modern cognitive semantics has to rely on the traditional meaning taxonomy to better understand the semantic networking of words. Therefore, when we analyze the disease metaphors in English and Chinese, we would include both novel metaphors and conventional conceptual metaphors that are less obvious but do play a critical role in our conceptualization of illness. In fact, the subconscious images employed in expressing illness or disease worth more attention in revealing the conventionalized schema in perceiving illness. Along with the development and prosperity of cognitive linguistics in the late 20th century, metaphor has proven to be a potent tool in deciphering human mind. It is treated as a fundamental approach in human cognition. That is, humans rely on metaphorical thinking to make sense of the surroundings more effectively. During our conceptualization of the world, metaphor is an indispensable tool in building connections between items and distilling information from the established connections, as well as in the construction and solidification of the conventionalized schema to facilitate future cognitive activities. Given metaphor's wide application in revealing the image schema in meaning construal and schematization, this book intends to use disease metaphors in Chinese and English to study people's perception of illness, with the hope of enhancing cross-cultural understanding as well as the varying countermeasures adopted by China and most English-speaking countries.

As mentioned above, the mental process includes four types: emotive, desiderative, perceptive and cognitive. If we argue that disease metaphors can reflect language user's view towards illness or diseases, we need to consider the view in a comprehensive way. That is, not only the meaning of disease metaphors should be studied, pragmatic factors like people's emotion, attitude towards the illness itself, patients, the causes and possible consequences of illness should also be taken into account. Generally speaking, emotive process denotes some feelings, giving a description of how people feel about something, which is usually expressed by words such as "like", "hate", "scare", "fear", "worry", "discourage", "comfort", "grieve" and so on. To understand the emotion in disease metaphors, in this book we rely on both the collocation analysis in corpus and the analysis of specific contexts of the random example sentences selected from the corpus. The semantic prosody of the frequent collocates of metaphor can provide us with a glimpse into the emotion involved in using certain disease metaphors. The same methods are also applied to better understand the desiderative process and the perceptive process. Different from the emotive process, the desiderative process describes the wishes and desires of people or personified objects, represented by verbs like "hope", "dream", "plan", "resolve", "covet", while the perceptive process is often presented by words such as "hear", "see", "smell", "witness", "look", "perceive" and so on, laying emphasis on the senses of human beings. The collocation analysis of disease metaphors that highlight the desiderative and perceptive processes can deepen our understanding of the attitude and perspective involved in the employment of certain metaphors. The last type of mental process concerned is the cognitive process, which describes the process by which human beings understand the world through psychological activities such as concept formation, perception, judgment or imagination. The cognitive process in clauses can often be reflected by verbs such as "understand", "forget", "realize", "dream", "expect", "strike", "remind" and "recall". The analysis of cognitive process through disease metaphors is mainly conducted on the basis of conceptual metphor theory, image schema and force dynamic theory. Different from emotive, desiderative and perceptive, it is hard to pin down specific verbs for cognitive process. Features of cognition are less obvious and usually underly the other mental processes, it is also more closely associated with life practice since the focus of attention, the perspectival mode adopted in cognitive scan, and the direction of the scanning are all embedded in daily lives, and are abstracted from real life practice.

Although the semantic configuration of these four processes are different, the main participants in the mental process are the same, namely, the Senser and the Phenomenon. In order to compare the conceptualization of illness or diseases between English and Chinese languages using metaphors, we combined the corpus-based analysis of metaphors and the qualitative metaphor analysis based on conceptual metaphor theory and image schema in establishing the semantic networks for "illness" in English and 病 in Chinese. Besides, we adopt event frame and force dynamics (Talmy, 2000) for further investigating people's emotion, attitudes towards illness, as well as the causes for illness or diseases.

The book consists of five chapters, which correspond to the five steps of the research process. In Chapter 1, we went through the previous related work that used metaphor to study meaning, culture and cognition. Both the systematic review of the representative studies and the quantative analysis of the prior research are conducted. In Chapter 2, guided by the semantic framework, we identified the first group of keywords to search for more data in general Chinese and English corpus, so as to further identify the main semantic themes commonly used in disease metaphors. To nail down the main themes used specifically in the accounts on diseases, we followed the MIVP approach in locating typical conceptual metaphors in self-established corpus of *China Daily* and BBC News. Further analysis of the contradictory themes from these two media is also carried out, and the frequent collocates of key words used in disease metaphors are visualized through the Word Sketch function in Sketch Engine. Chapters 3 and 4 mainly perform the qualitative analyses of disease metaphors in English and Chinese with the intention of understanding the cognitve schema and the influential social-cultural elements. In Chapter 3, we have carried out a detailed analysis of disease metaphors with plant images, with special attention paid to the "root/根" of a tree and the application of spatial-temporal schema in the formation of plant metaphors. Chapter 4 is mainly concerned with the understanding of causes of diseases in English and Chinese, highlighting the influence of social-cultural elements on the windowing of attention and the perspectives taken in viewing the causes for illness or diseases.

　　The innovation of this book lies in both its methods and the object of study. In terms of research methods, the book combines theory-based case analysis and corpus-based statistical analysis to provide a more convincing comparison for the understanding of diseases in English and Chinese. Besides, another innovative point in methods resides in the combination of the traditional lexicographical categorization of word meanings and the cogntive analysis of meaning extension. In this way, more dynamics can be introduced into the traditional categorization of word meanings, while the cognitive semantic analysis can be brought down to earth with a more systematic framework. Moreover, the current study is a comparative cognitive analysis of disease metaphors in English and Chinese, aiming to shed light on the emotive, perceptive and cognitive differences in understanding illness in English and Chinese, which can fill the gap in the cross-cultural cognitive analysis of metaphor. Apart from the innovation in methods, the research is using the up-to-date data for qualitative and quantative analysis. The self-established corpus is constructed using reports on China's handling of Covid-19 from *China Daily* and BBC News. Given the materials collected are concerned with the same topic, the contrastive analysis of disease metaphors used in the two corpus can serve as aptable materials for understanding the emotion, perception, position and cognition of diseases in English and Chinese. The study has both theoretical and practical values. The corpus-based cognitive and pragmatic analysis of disease metaphors provides a new comprehensive framework for investigating people's worldview through language, which is a more applicable framework in the study of the relationship between language and mind. As Saussure said, "Language is a system of symbols that condensed the wisdom of mankind. " In order to unveil the cognitive pattern through language, we need to supplement the contents that have been eliminated in the development of such a compact symbolic system, which include the emotion, position, attitude and social-cultural factors. That is why we need to enrich the framework used to analyze disease metaphors so as to gain better insights into the understanding of diseases in English and Chinese. As to the practical value, the comparative analysis of the cognitive, social-cultural reasons behind the choice of certain disease metaphors in English and Chinese can enhance the mutual understanding of diseases across cultures, which can lead to a higher degree of tolerance when people from difference culture perceive the same kind of illness differently, reduce possibility of the spreading of misinformation, and increases the chances of cross-cultural cooperation in coping with global pandemic like Covid-19. The construction of shared health community for mankind also relies on the precondition that different countries can have a better understanding of the conventionalized perceptual and cognitive pattern of diseases in another culture, especially when there are clear differences in viewing the causes, states and consequences of diseases.

Chapter 1

Metaphor as a Lens to Mind

The publication of *Metaphor We Live By* (Lakoff & Johnson, 1980) marks the beginning of wide-spreading studies on the cognitive functions of metaphors. The huge influence brought by Lakoff and Johnson's work has fundamentally changed the common classification of metaphors. In traditional linguistics, metaphor is considered as a figure of speech, which is mainly investigated in the branch of phraseology. However, along with the growing attention attributed to metaphor as a cognitive tool, it seems that metaphor and cognition are deeply combined. The mentioning of one would most definitely bring up the other.

The fast development of cognitive linguistics since the 1980s further accelerated the growing interest in metaphor study worldwide. Until now, there has been a stupendous amount of literature devoted to metaphor's role in human cognition. In this chapter, the author attempts to categorize the prior work into three groups. The first is generally concerned with the relationship between metaphor and cognition, in which different models to demonstrate metaphor's cognitive function will be introduced, such as the Idealized Conceptual Model (ICM) (Lakoff, 2008), the Image Schema (Langacker, 1987), as well as the mental space theory (Fauconnier & Turner, 1998). The second group is specifically devoted to metaphors' role in lexical meaning extension. In this part, different theories and models proposed by researchers to illustrate metaphor's function in lexical meaning extension will be introduced and compared. For example, the interactions between metaphor and metonymy in developing word meaning discussed in Littlemore's work will be summarized. And the interconnected model in word meaning extension proposed by Chinese researchers Wang & Wu (2020) and Shao & He (2012) will also be presented. Lexical

Chapter 1 Metaphor as a Lens to Mind

meaning extension is under the impact of both the cognitive and social factors. Conventionalized metaphors can be treated as the crystalization of both the cognitive pattern and social customs. Thus the study of metaphors provides us with a viable window to dissect the meaning formation, giving us a glimpse into the dynamic process.

This chapter will comb through the cross-cultural comparative cognitive studies through metaphor analysis. The curiosity about language's influence on human mind goes back to Humbolt (1999), and the degree of that influence is enlarged in Spair-Wholf hypothesis. Although there are controversy about the argument that language shapes people's way of thinking, more and more researchers tend to believe that language does exert a considerable amount of influence on people's thinking pattern. Just like many other behaviors of human beings, the way we think is also an outcome of conventionalization. That is to say, we, as human beings, habituate. Once we get used to certain behavior, we tend to follow the pattern, no matter it's a pattern of action, or a pattern of thinking.

If we agree that repeated movement will lead to a memory of the muscle, it should not be so difficult to consider the assumption that repeated usage of certain language patterns will also leave a dent or deepen the groove in our mind. Since language is mostly used in communication, the speech created by one speaker influences both the speaker and the listener, and for the sake of effective communication, only those wordings that can be understood by both interlocutors will be used repeatedly, increasing the possibility of being conventionalized.

Therefore, conventionalized metaphors can be seen as both the crystallization of thinking pattern and the conventionalization of social practice. Moreover, the thinking pattern and social practice are rather inter-wined than separated, which makes the pure study of semantic meaning without considering the pragmatic rules impossible (Cruse, 2004). Meanwhile, the fact that conventionalized metaphors can reflect both the cognitive process and social customs renders metaphor a potent approach in studying cultural characteristics of certain speech-community. In other words, metaphor not only provides us with a tangible window into how people think, it also demonstrates a potential path to understand how people behave in society, and maybe even why they behave in certain ways. With that being clarified, we can understand why more and more researchers are using metaphors to carry out cross-cultural studies.

1.1 Metaphor as a Way of Cognition

The idea that metaphor is human being's cognitive tool rather than a mere rhetoric is rooted in embodied philosophy. Different from transformation generative grammar of Chomsky (1978), embodied philosophy emphasizes the importance of daily practice in the development of our cognitive ability (Chen, 2006). Rather than believing the existence of a Language Acquisition Device (LAD), cognitive linguists are inclined to believe that human being's ability to use language is not an independent competence isolated from other cognitive abilities, but a part of the integrated human cognition. According to cognitive linguists, the cognitive domain activated when we use language is the same domain as employed in human being's other cognitive activities, which actually provides the precondition for studying the relationship between language acquisition and the development of human cognition. The claim that metaphor is an essential cognitive tool also emerges in this context.

Dating back to ancient Greek, metaphor means to "transfer or shift", which implies that metaphor, at the very beginning of its meaning construction, has a broader semantic scope. To put in simply, the ability to "metaphorize" is more or less equal to the ability to understand B through A based on the identified connections between A and B, and the connections are based on the similarity between them. In the process of human being's conceptualization of the world, naturally there is a sequence, in which things or concepts that are frequently applied in people's lives would be first entrenched in our minds, and things that are relatively less used or ideas above daily life practice would be internalized later. Then how can human beings move from concrete knowledge accumulated in daily experience to more abstract ideas? Or how can we understand things or concepts that are not directly rooted in our daily practice? For cognitive linguists, metaphor plays a pivotal role in this process, that is, in realizing the transfer or shift between the concrete ideas accessible in daily practice and the abstract concepts hanging above day-to-day practice (Lakoff & Johnson, 1980/2008).

Chapter 1 Metaphor as a Lens to Mind

The studies concerning metaphor's role in cognition can be roughly divided into three phases. The first phase is represented mainly by Lakoff and Johnson's seminal work—*Metaphors We Live By*, in which the concept of "domain mapping" was proposed. The term "domain" is similar to category, only that domain is limited to refer to the category of concepts rather than things. But we need to point out that studies on categorization can be dated back to Aristotle. As a matter of fact, many philosophers believe that the ability to categorize is one of human being's most fundamental ability. Therefore, it's fair to say that the term "domain" is developed on the basis of researches on categorization. By creating the term "domain mapping", Lakoff and Johnson constructed a simple explanation for how metaphor works in establishing the connections between different categories, especially in linking the concrete experiential knowledge to the abstract concepts. The idea is that when one can locate the common ground shared by different domains, a mapping can occur from the orginal domain that is more familiar to a person, to the target domain that is less familiar. The common ground usually refers to the similar features between the two domains. The typical example provided is Argument and War, in which War refers to the physical confrontation between two sides, and Argument is more of a verbal conflict between two sides. But since both Argument and War lay emphasis on the confrontation, conflicts in the process, and the winning or losing results in the end, words and phrases adopted in War description are commonly employed in illustrating Arguments between two sides. The "domain mapping" theory provides a simple interpretation for metaphor's function in connecting different categories. However, which features will be mapped and which will not are not specified. Besides, the motivation and steps in the realization of mapping is not explicated either.

The second phase is featured by Fauconnier's (1998) conceptual blending theory, which resolves the questioning about the uni-direction of mapping. The conceptual blending theory does not limit the connections between different categories into one or two directions. As a matter of fact, the blending theory is not concerned with the direction at all. The underlying logic for blending theory resembles the constructionist philosophy and coincides with the latest development in psychology, that is, meaning emerges from the blending of different elements rather than generated through purposeful repeated actions. Here we can notice that the term used by Fauconnier to refer to category is "mental space", which is more or less the same as Lakoff's "domain". But mental space attaches more importance to the spacial characteristics of human cognitive activities. Different from the simplicity and clarity of "domain mapping" theory, conceptual blending is more complicated and also ambiguous. The process of blending involves the construction of relations between different mental spaces in a conceptual integration network. The mental spaces include two or more input spaces, a generic space and a blended space. The main idea is that there would be selective mappings of elements occur among all the mental spaces, such as from generic spaces to input spaces, across input spaces, and from input spaces to the blend. At the first sight, the blending theory looks like an enhanced version of "domain mapping", only the mappings happen in a less ordered way between more spaces. And somehow the processes of this messy establishment of connections create emergent meaning.

It can be seen that the conceptual blending theory tries to capture the missed link in meaning generation process, which is not elaborated in the simple domain mapping scenario. The conceptual blending theory manages to bring the abstracted explanation closer to the more complicated and chaotic meaning construction process. However, the drawback is that the theory fails to provide guiding rules or principles in the multi-directional mappings between different spaces. Although the emergent meaning is an illuminating idea, the dynamic meaning constructing process still lurks in the darkness. We are certain that the process is definitely more complicated than simply domain mapping, but the establishment of complex interconnections between categories still remains under the dark water. We have no clue of how deep it is, and no anchor is provided to help us test or further explore.

Driven by the curiosity towards metaphor's role in cognition and the universal rules of human cognition in general, many cognitive linguists continued their efforts in explaining the century-old question about meaning formation. Enlightened by the development of modern psychology, various models have been proposed. Lakoff (1992) has furthered the domain mapping theory and presented the Idealized Cognitive Model (ICM). ICM is under the strong influence of the prototype theory in the studies of word meaning, the philosophy of which can be attributed to Wittgenstein's family resemblance hypothesis and game theory. The prototype theory argues that the meanings of words are not arranged in a well-organized list like a dictionary. Instead, wording meanings are grouped around prototypes. For each generic meaning, there would be a prototypical image in the center, and all the other similar images would revolve around the prototypical one. For example, for the category of fruit, the prototypical ones may be "apple", "pear" and "peach", in which "date" and "tomato" will be rather marginalized. Due to the different surroundings people live in, there may be different prototypes for the same category. Thus, the structure of each category and the boundary between categories can vary from culture to culture, which makes meaning formation under the heavy influence of sociocultural elements.

ICM goes hand in hand with Lakoff's conceptual metaphor theory, both imply that there exists a distilled abstract framework which overruns various types of specific metaphors. Guided by the conceptual metaphor, people tend to confine themselves to the restraints of ICM. It is like wearing a special pair of glasses, through which the world has already been generally categorized, and the initial idealized categorization and the entrenched connections between different categories serve as the model for further cognitive activities of human beings.

Another psychological theory that also accentuates the pattern or configuration one adopts in thinking is Gestalt theory that emerged in the early twentieth century in Austria and Germany (Koffka, 2013). Although Gestalt is primarily a psychological term, it has significant impact on the emergence of cognitive linguistics at the end of 20th century. Both Gestalt psychology and cognitive linguistics oppose atomism and are inclined to understand objects as an entire structure rather than the sum of its parts. The Gestalt psychologists emphasize that organisms perceive entire patterns or configurations, not merely individual components. The view is sometimes summarized using the adage "the whole is more than the sum of its parts". Similarly, cognitive linguistics also strive to unveil the pattern in cognitive activities, instead of treating the process of conceptualization as block-building. Many main theoretical frameworks in Gestalt psychology were borrowed into the cognitive analysis of languages. For example, the principle of reification, which highlights the generative aspect of perception, illuminates Lakoff's conceptual metaphor theory which relies on people's ability in imagining the contours of the analogical objects even when they are not shown or expressed directly. Besides, ICM also echoes with the principle of in-variance in

Gestalt psychology. The fact that ICM can guide various cognitive activities dates back to the invariance principle of perception, that is, people are able to recognize an object or event from different angles. Moreover, the principle of emergence is practically the same idea as Fauconnier's conceptual blending theory. The only difference is that emergence in psychology refers to the emerging properties or behaviors when the parts interact with a wider whole, while "emergent" is limited to describe meaning generated in mental spaces.

The most influential Gestalt principle in cognitive linguistics probably is the figure-ground perceptual organization. In psychology, figure-ground organization is the interpretation of perceptual elements in terms of their shapes and relative locations in the layout of surfaces in the 3-D world (Rubin, 2001). Figure-ground organization structures the perceptual field into a figure (standing out at the front of the perceptual field) and a background (receding behind the figure). The figure-ground contrast reveals both the unequal distribution of attention in viewing and the impact of perspective on cognition, which has shed light on the image schema theory of Langacker and Talmy's perspectival mode.

In the following part of this section, we will give a brief introduction to image schema and perspectival mode theory. As mentioned above, both of them are heavily influenced by Rubin's figure-ground perceptual organization principle. Langacker's image schema is featured by the visualization of conceptualization. By using simplified diagrams, Langacker attempts to illustrate the domain connection and meaning transfer using image schema. For example, Figure 1-1 shows the image schema for English verb "approach", from which we can see that trajector (tr) is visualized as an oval, and the landmark (lm) is illustrated as a target oval in another domain. The arrow in the following figure is employed to represent the trajectory for projection between various domains.

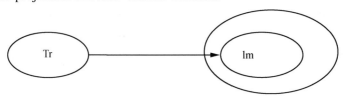

Figure 1-1 Image schema for "approach"

Langacker's image schema theory aims to conduct an anatomy of the meaning construction process, and those simplified symbols can help us clarify the major steps in meaning generation, paying special attention to the relationship establishment between different domains. Compared with the conceptual blending theory and ICM, image schema has taken a micro perspective, looking into the dynamic process of meaning construction. However, although the visual aids can indeed simplify the conceptualization, the drawback is that it can not capture the complicated influential factors in the sophisticated complex for meaning construction. Moreover, the choice of visual symbols used to illustrate domains and projections is to some extent subjective, which requires more evidence either from statistical corpus analysis or emperimental study of human brain and cognition. Besides, due to the rather static visualization of the cognitive activities, the dynamicity of meaning emergence can not be fully demonstrated.

Talmy's perspectival mode and force dynamic theory can compensate for the insufficiency of image schema. If we say that the image schema theory is constructed from an omniscient perspective, then the perspectival mode theory is viewing meaning generation from a person's eyes. The attention in perspectival mode is not paid to the hidden process of meaning formation, which is extremely difficult for us to explore without building preliminary conclusions on a series of rather subjective assumptions, just like the image shema theory. Whether it is right or wrong still hangs in the air, waiting to be confirmed with new breakthroughs either in psychological study or brain science. On the contrary, the perspectival mode theory believes that the magic happens outside the brain. Associations between cognitive domains and the rule for categorization are not the major concern here. The stress is laid on the viewer. That is, the viewer's orientation in space, the scope and direction of cognitive scanning affect the viewer's observation, leading to different meaning construction. Instead of viewing the meaning formation as an enclosed process with clear boudaries, Talmy dates back to the basic senses needed in meaning formation, especially visuality.

The perspectival mode theory is in line with other main theoretical framework discussed in his two volumes of cognitive semantics, including the "fictive motion", the "windowing of attention", and the force dynamics in language and cognition. Talmy seeks to account for expressions that depict motion when there is no physical occurence of motion: "This fence goes from the plateau to the valley"; "The cliff faces toward/away from the island"; "I looked out past the steeple"; "The vacuum cleaner is down around behind the clothes-hamper"; "The scenery rushed past us as we drove along". The direction and scope of scanning as well as the view point included in perspectival mode are dependant on the fictive motion of one's sight. Besides, the perspectival mode is also related to the windowing of attention, that is, what lies in the viewer's attention focus and what is gapped or backgrounded. Be aware that what's been gapped does not mean that they are not receiving any attention. The gap only indicates relatively less amount of attention compared with the focus. Meanwhile, the relationship between gap and the window is similar to that between ground and figure. The windowing can not be realized without the gapping.

In summary, it can be seen that in the cognitive study metaphor is inalienable from the study of meaning formation or generation. From the simple domain mapping theory, to blending, then to image schema, force dynamics, and perspectival mode, all of the theoretical frameworks aim to clarify the process of meaning formation. Different from Chomsky's influential transform-generative grammar, cognitive linguists are convinced that the study of the pure form of language leads to nowhere. A deeper understanding of language and human cognition can not be realized unless the meaning of language is taken into account. Meaning formation and language development go hand in hand, and the key to resolve the mystery of language can only be found in the interface between meaning and form.

1.2 Metaphor's Role in Lexical Meaning Extension

Under the wide-spread influence of Chomsky's universal grammar concept, a large number of linguists attach importance only to functional grammatical words and phrases. Although the work of the cogntive linguists like Lakoff, Langacker and Talmy has drawn more attention to the study of meaning, the meaning study is limited to the meaning of grammatical structure, for example, the meaning of constructions (Goldberg, Brown & Miller, 1996), and the meaning of functional words (Langacker, 1987). Few studies are devoted to the investigation of lexical words. There may be three main reasons for the lack of interest in the study of lexical word meanings. First, the ambition of modern linguits is to reveal the relationship between language and mind, thus the common cognitive competence of mankind is what they are concerned with. Since lexical words are so diversified in meaning, and are largely dependent on the language as well as cultural context in certain language community, it would be extremely hard for the researchers to pinpoint some common rules or principles in human cognition. Therefore, naturally, functional words or grammatical structures that are more or less universal in all kinds human languages seem like a feasible approach to understanding the mutual influence between language and mind. The second reason for the reluctance in researching lexical word meaning is mainly concerned with the mere difficulty. As mentioned in the first reason, lexical meaning is context-dependant, which makes it ambiguous and less delicate. Compared with form, meaning is already a challenging task to begin with. The meaning of lexical word is even more difficult to grasp and identify. It is easy to get lost in the ocean of lexical meanings and forget about the original intention, which is to seek pattern out of the meaning, so we can connect the word meaning with the cognitive meaning, thus having a deepened understanding of forms. However, due to the sheer volume and higher degree of uncertainty, it is notoriously hard to discover the track beneath the behemoth amount of water, especially when the corpus technology is not yet well established in the late 20th or the early 21th century. The third reason for the little progress accomplished in the cogntive study of lexical words probably goes to the requirement of encyclopedic cross-disciplinary knowledge for digging out the reasons for the meaning extension of lexical words and phrases. The reasons for the meaning evolvement of lexical words is influenced by many scattered factors. It would be really challenging for an individual researcher to collect all the pieces to complete the whole puzzle.

  Therefore, due to the above three reasons, studies of lexical meaning are left behind compared with the meaning investigation of grammatical structure and words. The same trend can also be found among domestic scholars who have shown interest in the study of meaning. For example, Liu & Li (2020) still upholds the philosophy that the exploration of human cognition and the conceptualization of the world should attach importance to grammatical or functional words rather than lexical words. He believes that the meaningful meaning can only be obtained in structure rather than nodes. As a matter of fact, this philosophy has deep historic echoes. It can date back to the early distinction between *parole* and *langua* of Sausurre, and the more recent separation between performance and competence, as well as semantics and syntax. It's like admitting that meaning can influence form, but do not want to accept that all kinds of meanings are capable of playing a role in shaping form. Thus we need to stratify meaning into structural meaning, like that of functional words and grammatical structure, and the less organized meaning, like that of lexical words. However, if we are saying that meaning formation is a dynamic process, and as cognitive semanticist argued, there exists an idealized model or schema in meaning formation or generation, then why the only way to prove the existence of such a model or schema is to look for the model in all kinds of meanings rather than only in the selected structural meanings. Therefore, the author believes that the study of lexical meaning is also highly relevant to the journey toward human cognition. Furthermore, what can not be discovered in the typological analysis of grammar and structure can be compensated by the detailed cross-language investigation of the lexical word meaning formation.

In the late 20th century, along with the further development of psychology and neuroscience, more empirical evidence in favor of the hypothesized ICM or image schema has been discovered. It seems that different places of human brain are activated in the use of language rather than a particular spot in brain. Besides, people who can not speak well due to brain damage are able to regain and improve their language skills through persistent enhanced practice designed to train certain linguistic competence, which makes people question the existence of an innate language acquisition device in human brain. Besides, the psychological evidence that people tend to be attracted by moving things, the highlighted figure in the ground seems to be in line with the formation of metaphor in language, which also requires selective projection. This also proves that language is not an isolated compentence controlled by a specific area of human brain, but rather resides in the common cognitive ability of human beings.

Apart from the favorable psychological and neuroscience evidence, the path towards the understanding of human cognition and the meaning of language is made less daunting with the development of corpus technology. The advance of corpus technology has facilitated the identification of underlying pattern among seemly diversified and ambiguous meaning evolution. Equipped with corpus tool, it is much less time-consuming to reveal the tendency in collocation, the semantic prosody in frequent collocates, as well as the distribution of words in different themes, providing an edge in exploring the dynamic meaning formation in its dynamicity.

Since the 1980s, more and more linguists have turned their attention towards the meaning of words, leading to the maturity of lexical semantics as an independent direction in cognitive linguistics. As one of the pioneers in studying lexical semantics, Fillmore (1976) brought forward the concept of "frame semantics" in an attempt to systematize the diversified meanings of words and to provide unified interpretation for the relationship between different meaning items and reasons for meaning evolution. However, instead of focusing on the meaning of content words, frame semantics is mainly concerned with functional words and grammatical structures. Cruse (2004) and Taylor (1993) continued the line of lexical semantics by looking at different types of functional words, such as comparatives and prepositions, and some synonymous and antonymous words and expressions. Due to the fact that corpus technology is less developed at that time, most of the explanations of content words are limited to qualitative analysis, relying much on the induction and deduction of the authors with a few example sentences as illustration. The lack of quantitative analysis makes the interpretation of content word meaning less convincing and unsustainable.

Influenced by the growing interest in lexical semantics, quite a few domestic researchers have started to decipher human cognition through word meaning analysis. Similar to the path taken by foreign researchers, domestic linguists also started with functional words and grammatical structures. There emerged a large number of studies concerning the Chinese auxiliary verb "ba" (Huang, 2014; Wu & Tian, 2018; Zhang, 2020), the adjective marker "de", the aspect marker "le", and other functional words as well as grammatical constructions. Apart from the attention to functional words, some researchers also tried to depict the model for the meaning extension of content words. The most frequent approach in the exploration of diachronic meaning evolution of words is through the analysis of metaphors and metonymy. It is acknowledged that metaphor plays an essential role in meaning extension (Sweester, 1999), yet how exactly metaphorical projection influences meaning formation is not clear. Besides, we are aware that metaphorical projection is based on the similarities between the source and target domains. We also know that the projection only selects and highlights some features of the source domain. Then the question lies in which features to select and why, since the similarities we see from two domains may vary if we assume different perspectives. The exploration of the reasons behind the accustomed feature selection and the conventionalized perspective gives us a hint on how human beings conceptualize their surroundings.

The consecutive metaphorical projection towards certain direction results in the meaning extension of the words. Wang & Wu (2020) proposed a cactus-shaped model to demonstrate the interconnection between different rounds of domain mapping. The shape of the connected or overlapped domain resembles that of a cactus. The cactus-shaped model to demonstrate metaphor's role in extending word meaning provides us with a simplified and static overview of the possible meaning extension. However, it fails to capture the reasons for the tendency towards certain direction. That is why the cactus grows in this particular shape. The reason behind the direction of growing and the interconnection between different chunks of the cactus is unclear. Since the cross-domain mapping is based on the selected features of certain cognitive domains, then what is the reason for selecting a particular group of features instead of others? In other words, what is behind the windowing and gaping, or what determines the delineation of figure and ground? Those questions are largely left unanswered. The fact that the reasons behind the selection are not well explored is understandable, since the investigation of the underlying reasons behind the differentiation between figure and ground seems to be a topic within psychology rather than linguistics. However, if we want to make more progress in understanding the relationship between language and human cognition, to carry out cross-disciplinary study is the only true answer. Especially for psycholinguistics and neurolinguistics, both of them attempt to clarify the relationship between language and human cognition. In terms of metaphor's role in meaning extension, psycholinguistics aims to answer the question by studying people's behavior, while neurolinguistics focuses on how human mind works.

Therefore, despite the efforts made in exploring metaphor's role in meaning extension, there still remain questions to be answered. This book attaches more importance to the psycho-linguistic approach in dealing with the question, paying more attention to the influence of conventionalized practice on meaning interpretation. In other words, we intends to explain the semantic evolution of words from a pragmatic perspective.

1.3 Cross-Cultural Cognitive Studies through Metaphors

The best way to learn about how people from certain language community think and behave is through comparison. Through comparison, the distinguished features of one language community can be highlighted and the universal nature in cognition across different cultures and communities can be revealed. Besides, the comparison about the use of certain metaphors in different languages and cultures can provide us with a deeper understanding of metaphor's role in meaning extension as well as the common cognitive principle shared by different languages and cultures.

In the 1980s and 1990s, lexical semantics gradually matured (Fillmore, 1976; Cruse, 2004; Talyor, 1993), focusing on the association between lexical items and the cognitive process of lexical meaning. At the beginning of the 20th century, cognitive semantics started to pay more attention to the meaning evolution at the vocabulary level. The meaning evolution of a particular basic word in one language can provide us with a window to understand the meaning construction from a diachronic perspective. However, most of the previous work in the international academic is limited to the research on English vocabulary (Taylor, 2003; Coulson, 2001). Few studies have paid attention to the lexical meaning evolution in other languages. Under the influence of the growing interest in the lexical meaning abroad, the domestic lexical research has also increasingly focused on the cognitive meaning construction of words.

However, as far as the target language is concerned, domestic studies on lexical meaning are mostly limited to Chinese (Dai & Ye, 1990; Zhang, 1994), with few comparative studies between Chinese and English vocabulary. From the late 20th century to the early 21st century, lexical semantic studies at home and abroad were roughly divided into two perspectives: first, the diachronic study, which emphasizes on the role of metaphor and metonymy in the derivation of word meanings (Sweetser, 1990; Lin & Yang, 2005) and the construction of meaning derivation models (Xiong, 2011; Wang, 2015); second, the synchronic study, which focuses on the syntactic-semantic interface, explaining the cognitive causes of lexical ambiguity through the construction of universal cognitive grammar (Goldberg, 1995a/1995b; Lu, 2004; Yuan & Wang, 2002). However, there are relatively fewer studies devoted to the cross-cultural comparison of lexical-semantic networks of words with similar basic meaning that combine the two perspectives.

In fact, synchronic study can provide a more comprehensive framework of word meaning through the analysis of correlates, which is conducive to further investigating of the meaning evolution from a diachronic angle. Meanwhile, diachronic analysis of word meaning provides an explanation for the current meaning network of word. Therefore, it is of significance to combine the two perspectives in the investigation of word meaning development.

At the beginning of the 21st century, there was a "social turn" in the international study of lexical meaning. More and more researchers of lexical semantics realized the importance of context and the social-historical factors in word meaning development, which advocated the re-contextualization in the cognitive studies of word meaning (Coulson, 2001; Cruse, 2004). Besides, also in the first period of the 21th century, the development of psychology and the maturation of corpora has provided further momentum for the "empirical turn" in studying lexical meaning, leading to more corpus-based lexical cognition studies (Goddard & Wierzbicka, 2013). In the last decade, Chinese researchers have also started to use corpus statistics to reveal the meaning distribution of words and the characteristics of cognition (Shao & He, 2012; Liu & Li, 2020), but the overall number of studies is still small and there is a lack of attention on social dimension.

In the following chapters, we will construct the semantic network for both correspondent words related to "illness" in English and words relevant to 病 in Chinese. By establishing the semantic networks for "illness" and 病, we would be able to have a more comprehensive understanding of how illness/病 is perceived in China and the English-speaking countries. Besides, we will carry out more detailed comparison between metaphors of "illness" and metaphors of 病 with different kinds of images, such as natural images and super natural images. Illness-related metaphors with ethnomedical concepts will be compared too. Based on the comparative analysis of illness-related metaphors in both English and Chinese, we would be able to identify the similarities and differences in the overall perception of illness in China and in the English-speaking world. In addition, we will discuss social-cultural evidence and reason to justify and explain how these similarities and differences are formed, deepening our understanding of the domestic and foreign views toward illness.

The study employs quantitative and qualitative analysis. Corpus searching results are used to corroborate the preliminary conclusion through comparative analysis of disease metaphors. Besides, visualization method is adopted to present the structural similarities and differences between the semantic network of Chinese 病 and English "illness", which can give us a bird's-eye view of the perception of illness China and the English-speaking countries.

During the Covid-19 pandemic, there have been conflictory opinions about how human beings should handle the disease. The different policies adopted by governments across the world have been heavily politicized. Misunderstanding and mis-interpretation hampered the sharing of effective measures in preventing the virus from spreading, which has led to undesirable results. Despite the ideological difference, the lack of mutual understanding in the common perception of illness in different language communities also plays a part in deteriorating the misunderstanding and accelerating the spreading of misinformation. Against this background, the comparative analysis of disease metaphors in English and Chinese is especially valuable in today's world, for it can help people of different language communities and from different backgrounds to shift perspectives and understand how illness is perceived from the other side of the world. Equiped with a more inclusive understanding of illness, people's mindset and attitude towards illness can become more inclusive too, thus paving the way for the establishment of a healthy community with shared future of mankind.

1.4 Bibliometric Analysis of Studies on Disease Metaphors

Ever since Lakoff and Johnson's phenomenal work *Metaphors We Live By*, there has emerged a tremendous amount of work devoted to conceptual metaphors. Among them, disease metaphors only take up a relatively small share.

In this section, we use two bibliometric softwares to help us develop a overview of the prior work on disease metaphors. In order to better understand the previous work, and identify the recent up-to-date research focuses, we have searched for "disease" and "metaphor" in the Web of Science core collection—Social Science Citation Index from 1900 to present. After filtering, we have located more than 500 articles on this theme. Then we downloaded the full records and references of the articles, and visualized the prior work on disease metaphors through VOSviewer, so as to locate the main research fields when it comes to disease metaphors. Besides, we also input the data into CitNetExplorer to identify the hot topics in this field. The following figure demonstrates the co-occurrences of keywords in the published articles. It can be seen from Figure 1-2 that "cancer", "communication", "dementia", "alzheimer's disease" are the keywords that occur more frequently besides the most relevant keywords like "metaphor", "disease" and "health". Those keywords indicate two main lines of research about disease metaphor. The first line concerns studies that intend to use metaphor as a way to treat patients with syndromes related to the degeneration of brain, including diseases like "dementia" and "alzheimer's disease". Metaphor has been proved to be a potentially effective approach to stimulate and enhance the re-growth of synapse of neurons, that's why many clinics around the world are using specially designed language materials full of metaphors to treat patients with similar brain diseases. The second line of research is mainly reflected through the keyword "communication", which is about the role metaphor plays in medical discourse between doctors and patients. Proper use of metaphors in medical discourse can facilitate the diagnosing process and avoid misunderstanding, while inappropriate use of metaphors might result in unpleasant conversations or even conflicts between doctors and patients. However, these two lines of research on disease metaphor are not directly concerned with people's cognition of disease, or metaphor's role in assisting us in conceptualizing disease or illness. These two lines of research pay more attention to the pragmatic analysis of metaphors or the practical application of metaphors in medical treatment rather than investigating metaphor's role in cognition.

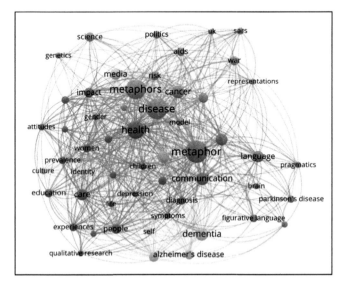

Figure 1-2 Visualization of co-occurrences of keywords in disease metaphor studies

The only keyword in Figure 1-2 that indicates the study about the formation of disease metaphor is "war", which is not a very big node on the upper right area of the figure. "DISEASE IS WAR" is indeed a common conceptual metaphor in both English and Chinese. It is common to think of the frequent verbal collocates when it comes to disease, such as "fight with the disease", or 与疾病作斗争 in Chinese. In both phrases, disease is seen as the enemy, and our immune system is the soldier who would fight with the enemy to protect our health. However, apart from the "war metaphor", we can hardly find any illuminating keywords that can provide us with more information about the metaphorical images we may use in conceptualizing diseases. The lack of keywords directly related to disease metaphors in the co-occurrence map also demonstrates that the study of conceptual disease metaphors within the framework of cognitive linguistics is still insufficient.

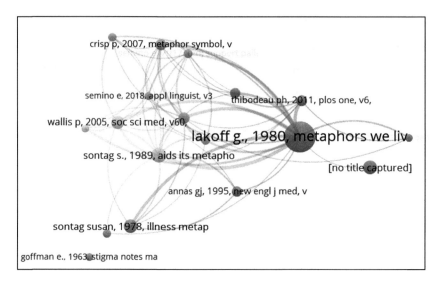

Figure 1-3 Visualization of top 10 academic publications with the highest co-citations

We set the minimum number of citations of cited reference at 12, by using VOSviewer we obtained from the above figure, which displays the top 10 academic publications on disease metaphor in terms of the number of co-citations. We can see from Figure 3 that the biggest circle goes to Lakoff & Johnson's *Metaphor We Live By*. Besides, there are four publications before 1990s, including Susan's work in 1978 about illness metaphor, which is the earliest literature shown in this figure. In the book *Illness as a Metaphor*, Susan carried out a critical analysis of the discourse on illness between doctors and patients, so as to relieve the patient of being the one deserving criticism. Susan's work can be regarded as one of the earliest contributions to the discourse analysis approach in metaphor study. This line of research is more closely associated with the pragmatic study of metaphors, emphasizing metaphor's role in identity construction. The recent publications about disease metaphor were contributed by Elena Semino, who has written several articles about disease metaphor based on corpus searching results. Two of her most recent publications have discussed metaphors employed in describing "cancer" and "Covid-19". The article published in *Applied Linguistics* provides an integrated approach to metaphor and framing in cognition, discourse, and practice, which can serve as a functional approach in the study of metaphor from different perspectives, including both social and cognitive angles. The most recent paper published in *Health Communication* brought a new angel in visualizing the doctors during the pandemic. Different from the traditional war metaphors, she brought up the "firefighter" metaphor based on the corpus, which painted a more dynamic picture of the ongoing emergency during the pandemic. More researches on disease metaphor can be found in the following table, from which we can find that studies about disease metaphor are mainly published in four kinds of journals: journals that focus on the medical discourse like *Health Communication* and *Journal of Communication*; journals about the relationship between language competence and human brain, such as *Brain Language*; journals that focus on medicines like *Social Science Medicine*, *New English Journal of Medicine*, and *Journal of Clinic Oncology*; journals interested in metaphor studies and linguistics in general, such as *Metaphor Symbol* and *Applied Linguistics*.

Table 1-1 Ranking of the publications on disease metaphor based on citation numbers

No.	Publications	Links	Total Link Strength	Citations
1	lakoff g., 1980, metaphors we live	18	178	101
2	sontag s., 1989, aids its metaphors	15	98	32
3	sontag susan, 1978, illness metaphor	14	46	29
4	wallis p, 2005, soc sci med	15	64	26
5	gibbs rw, 2002, health commun	15	87	21
6	crisp p, 2007, metaphor symbol	13	77	20
7	thibodeau ph, 2011, plos one	14	55	19
8	annas gj, 1995, new engl j med	11	29	18
9	entman rm, 1993, j commun	14	42	18
10	reisfield gm, 2004, j clin oncol	14	56	15
11	semino e, 2017, bmj support palliat	14	67	15
12	braun v., 2006, qualitative res psyc	11	18	13
13	semino e, 2021, health commun	11	38	13
14	amanzio m, 2008, brain lang	3	8	12
15	charterisblack j, 2004, corpus approaches to critical metaphor analysis	13	39	12

(continuous)

No.	Publications	Links	Total Link Strength	Citations
16	gibbs r. w, 1994, poetics mind figurat	13	31	12
17	goffman e., 1963, stigma notes managem	2	2	12
18	semino e, 2018, appl linguist	14	47	12
19	winner e, 1977, brain	2	8	12

  Metaphor is simple due to that it originates in the intrinsic analogical thinking of human beings, and it is formed simply by connecting one thing to another. At the same time, it is complicated in that there are so many diversified ways of selection of features and directions for projection. Metaphor is like neurons. It connects and sends messages to the brain to help us better understand ourselves and the world around us. Although like neurons, metaphor is simple in its internal structure or components, metaphor's magic lies in the connection between things, and the linking is where its power resides. Just like neurons, one neuron can hardly do anything, but when the number is big enough, there is hardly anything it can not accomplish.

  This book intends to compare disease metaphors commonly used in English and Chinese, with an intention to provide a bigger picture of how disease can be perceived and understood. We usually take what is in our culture for granted. Only through comparison can we become more aware of the assumptions and the underlying conceptual metaphors we adopt in seeing and interpreting the surroundings and what is happening in the world.

Chapter 2

Corpus-Based Comparison of Disease Metaphors in English and Chinese

Metaphor is at essence the analogy between two things with similar features, which plays a fundamental role in human's conceptualization of the surroundings (Lakoff & Johnson, 1980/2008). People start to understand the world during their daily practice. They construct the network of knowledge and meaning from their interactions with things they can get in touch with, and events they can experience. Then they would project their knowledge and experience of the things they are familiar with to the other domains that are either far away from their daily practice or too abstract and complicated to comprehend.

Given the similarity in the environment we live in and the common physical conditions of human beings, people from different parts of the world have developed metaphors based on similar natural images or common life practice. Among them, metaphors with natural images, especially plants, are widespread in many different cultures, including English and Chinese.

In this chapter, we will compare metaphors with the same or similar source domain in English and Chinese languages. By comparing the target domains adopted for the same source domain, we can gain a clearer understanding of people's conceptualization of the source domain in English and Chinese. Disease is a prevalent phenomenon in different cultures, and it is rather elusive and terrifying in the primitive stage of human civilization. In ancient times, people may attribute diseases to supernaturalism, especially infectious diseases like plague or pandemic. Besides, diseases are also analyzed using familiar objects or events in people's daily practice.

In order to better depict the reason, process and results of disease, people from different cultures may rely on images from nature. For example, in many cultures people compare human life to the growth of a tree. Many life-related metaphors thus are using the features of trees as the source domain. As one of the obstacles in human life, many disease metaphors also gain inspirations from the characteristics of a tree or a plant. Apart from tree or plant metaphors, LIFE IS A JOURNEY and LIFE IS A RIVER are also common conceptual metaphors existed in both English and Chinese. In this chapter, we will mainly analyze disease metaphors with natural images as the source domain and compare the formation of these kinds of disease metaphors between English and Chinese. Besides, we also intend to investigate the cognitive and social reasons for the similarities and differences in the selection of features and in the projection between domains.

Before we look into disease metaphors using natural images, we will first identify the metaphorical themes of disease-related data using Wmatrix. The steps of data analysis are as follows: (1) search for illness-related words in BNC, and download the random samples from the searching results of each word, including "illness, disease, ailment and medical condition"; (2) search for 病 related characters in online Chinese corpus of Sketch engine, and download the random samples from the search results of every character, including 病, 疾, 恙, 疴 and 疫; (3) upload the English and Chinese data into Wmatrix, and identify the main metaphorical themes of the materials; (4) identify the specific metaphors within each theme following the procedures of MIVPU; (5) compare the metaphorical themes between English and Chinese, and analyze the specific metaphors to support the conclusion.

2.1 Corpus-Based Comparison of Semantic Themes of Disease Metaphors in English and Chinese

In this section, using corpus analysis, the semantic structure of "disease" in English and Chinese is compared, as well as the main metaphorical themes in news report on Covid in BBC News and *China Daily*. Besides, the distribution features of typical disease metaphors in the established corpus of *China Daily* and BBC News are also discussed. In addition, a further reason analysis of the contradictory themes and a visualization of the key disease metaphors are also included.

2.1.1 Comparison of the Semantic Themes of the Collocates of "Illness" and "Disease"

With the semantic tagging of Wmatrix, we were able to identify the main conceptual themes used in describing "illness" and "disease". In the following tables of this section we can find that "illness" and "disease" do share several themes in common, yet the priority of the themes differ. For example, both "illness" and "disease" share the theme that "Illness or disease is danger", while the theme "Danger" ranked as No. 4 frequent theme according to Logliklihood, for "disease" "Danger" only ranked as No. 12 theme for "illness", which proves our preliminary deduction, that is, compared with illness, disease tends to be more serious, acute and life-threatening. Another theme "disease" and "illness" share in common is "Illness or disease is hindering", or we may say that "illness" or "disease" can be seen as the "obstacle" or "barrier" in one's life journey. Despite the fact that both "illness" and "disease" have this semantic theme "hindering", "hindering" enjoys a higher status in the semantic themes of "disease" than it does in the themes of "illness". The fact that "disease" is more likely to be viewed as "hindering" than "illness" is rooted in similar reasons, that is, disease is usually more severe, thus would be more disruptive in one's daily life.

Apart from these two themes, the fact that "Mental actions and processes" ranks as the third most frequent theme of "illness" echoes our comparison between the semantic scope between "illness" and "disease", that is, nowadays "illness" in English tends to be used more to refer to mental medical problems. On the contrary, the third theme for "disease" is "Anatomy and physiology", proving our analysis that "disease" is more closely associated with medical problems that concern human organs. Another interesting thing to notice in the ranking of the semantic themes between "illness" and "disease" is that, although "disease" is more frequently connected to "Danger", "illness" is the word that reminds people of "Dead", "Sad" and "Bad evaluation". Besides, the "people" theme also rank higher on the side of "illness" despite the fact that "disease" is the one that directly relates to human bodies. All of these suggest that "illness" is more about "soul", while "disease" is concerned with "body". "Illness" enjoys more negative pragmatic color than "disease", in other words, "disease" is closer to the neutral and objective medical terms, while "illness" is the word that is closer to human life. That explains why themes like "Dead, alive, people" all ranked higher in "illness". On the side of "disease", we see more themes related to medical science. For example, themes like "Science and technology", "Investigate, examine, test" as well as "Substances and materials" are the high-ranking themes, demonstrating the objectivity and professional nature of "disease".

Apart from the relevant high-ranking semantic themes listed above, we can also identify some uncommon themes in both "illness" and "disease" which are used more frequently when we place these two groups of mini-corpora against the BNC written sample. For "illness", after filtering through the usual themes (Table 2-1), we fail to identify obvious metaphorical projections across domains. The reason that there is hardly any metaphor in the semantic themes of "illness" probably goes to the fact that "illness" is very closely inter-wined with human lives and is deeply integrated into daily practice. Instead of being the target domain, "illness" is more likely to be used as the source domain in the conceptualization of the world.

The main semantic themes of "illness" listed in Table 2-1 also support our argument. We can see that apart from the obvious themes related to disease, medicines and health, the high-ranking themes are very much involved in daily life practice, which makes "illness" less likely to be described in a metaphorical way.

Table 2-1 Main semantic themes of the collocation of "illness"

No.	Item	O1	%1	O2	%2	LL	%DIFF	Semantic Themes
1	B2 −	1791	6.48	1275	0.13 +	8748.30	4821.41	Disease
2	B3	478	1.73	1711	0.18 +	1225.38	878.77	Medicines and medical treatment
3	X2	186	0.67	46	0.00 +	1104.95	14066.39	Mental actions and processes
4	B2	83	0.30	129	0.01 +	318.45	2154.20	Health and disease
5	S2	273	0.99	2896	0.30 +	259.73	230.27	People
6	A2.2	326	1.18	4362	0.45 +	215.68	161.84	Cause & Effect/Connection
7	L1 −	169	0.61	1585	0.16 +	188.77	273.56	Dead
8	L1 +	42	0.15	93	0.01 +	138.94	1482.23	Alive
9	T1.3 +	95	0.34	733	0.08 +	132.28	354.07	Time period: long

(continuous)

No	Item	O1	%1	O2	%2	LL	%DIFF	Semantic Themes
10	E4.1 −	107	0.39	979	0.10 +	123.16	282.92	Sad
11	A15 −	58	0.21	370	0.04 +	97.02	449.20	Danger
12	S8 +	238	0.86	4225	0.44 +	85.65	97.3	Helping
13	A5.1 −	69	0.25	624	0.06 +	80.54	287.41	Evaluation: bad
14	B2 +	28	0.10	195	0.02 +	43.18	403.07	Healthy
15	S8 −	63	0.23	885	0.09 +	38.13	149.40	Hindering
16	H4 −	7	0.03	10	0.00 +	27.71	2352.46	Non-resident
17	B1	221	0.80	5489	0.57 +	22.67	41.06	Anatomy and physiology
18	A1.1.	247	0.17	815	0.08 +	17.97	102.04	Damaging and destroying
19	F3	15	0.05	135	0.01 +	17.61	289.28	Smoking and non-medical drugs

Although there is no evident metaphor employed in the description of "illness", we did notice some themes that are closely associated with "illness", including "Alive", "Time" "Long period", "Sad", "Danger" and "Damaging power", which can further our understanding of how "illness" is perceived in English. Several example sentences from the online English web2020 corpus of the Sketch Engine platform within each of these three themes are listed as follows:

- **Alive**

St. 1　I have personal experience of the way mental **illness** can wreck your **life Alive**.

St. 2　Co-author David Christiani did however note in a statement that he doesn't believe the glucan levels are linked to the mysterious "vaping **illness**" that has claimed the **lives** of more than 50 people as of December.

- **Sad**

St. 3　Mental **illnesses** such as **depression** and anxiety often co-occur with substance abuse.

St. 4　Harry Lovelock, Mental Health Australia Director, said the income allowance is "inadequate" and taking an unfair toll on those **suffering mental illnesses**.

- **Danger**

St. 5　However, the FDA found that there were sufficient grounds for removing ephedrine-containing drugs from the marketplace because they presented "**unreasonable risk of illness** or injury".

St. 6　They also face an increased **risk of chronic illness** during adulthood.

- **Long**

St. 7　Park C. Woodyard, 87, of Shock, Gilmer County, died Feb. 20, 1997, in Braxton County Memorial Hospital, Gassaway, after a **long illness**.

- **Damaging, destroying power**

St. 8　Students with physical disabilities, neurologically based disorders which trigger a physical response, students **disabled** by a chronic **illness** and have physical complications due to that illness.

St. 9　She is now the leader of the HIV/TB Center within IDM, building mathematical models of HIV and TB to understand how to robustly and rapidly reduce incidence and deaths from these two **devastating illnesses**.

After the analysis of typical sentence, we can summarize the part of the perceived features of "illness" in English from the above example sentences, together with the semantic themes listed in Table 2-1. Illness is usually seen as a relatively long process in human lives, which is able to make us suffer, especially mentally. It is the risk in life we are not willing to take, and the danger we all try to avoid and prevent.

In addition, it is shown in Table 2-1 that the evaluation of illness is one of the high-ranking themes, and the general evaluation of "illness" is not surprisingly negative. From this theme we can also learn about people's cognition and attitude towards the word "illness". That is, when "illness" is used, the interlocutors are usually not keen to learn about what is the illness exactly, or what are the medical reasons, or the syndromes for the "illness", in other words, the mentioning of the word "illness" dost not arouse people's desire to investigate, examine or test. Instead, the word "illness" triggers more "depressive" emotion and "dislike" in attitude. The expression of emotional and attitudinal value is strong in the word "illness". For example, one interesting theme of "illness" is "Non-resident", which is associated with homeless people. For example,

- **Non-resident**

St. 10　TPCH says nearly 1,500 people are **homeless** as of January 2018 and nearly half of them suffer from substance abuse disorder or **mental illness**.

St. 11 Service goals include the prevention of exacerbation of a condition, preventing injury to the person served or others, providing treatment in the context of the least restrictive setting, averting or reducing the threat of inpatient psychiatric hospitalization, incarceration, or **homelessness**, and assessing and stabilizing acute **symptoms of mental illness**, **alcohol** and other **substance abuse**.

It can be seen from the two example sentences of "Non-resident" theme of "illness" that the collocates or words that tend to co-occur with "illness" are largely negative. Here the negative is not just about being ill itself, but also suggests the common semantic association for "illness". Since "illness" is more about the general depiction of being in an unhealthy state, it tends to correlate with other undesirable condition like "poverty", "homelessness", as well as possible personal reasons for being ill. Unlike "disease", the wording about which is neutral and objective, "illness" is negative in attitude values, including both evaluation and judgement. People studies "disease" and try to cure "disease", while we dislikes "illness" and try to drive away "illness".

The fact that "Non-resident" theme is one of the common semantic themes of "illness", but not of "disease" also supports our analysis, that is, "illness" tends to go hand in hand with other unwanted things and events, such as "poverty", "abuse", "low self-control", etc. It seems that when one is ill, we either feel sorry for him or her, or think he or she probably deserves it for not leading a healthy life. However, when we say that someone has contracted a kind of disease, the most common response is either being empathetic or being curious about the syndromes or the cure of the disease. The stylistic distinction between "illness" and "disease" actually provides a rational zone which filters people's emotional fear or dislike, and helps to maintain a rational attitude towards those who are infected with "disease". Meanwhile, there is no clear boundary between the Chinese equivalent for "illness" and "disease", namely, 病 and 疾. Could the lack of semantic borderline between 病 and 疾 also blur people's feeling and attitude towards people who become 病 and those who are infected by 疾? We will further analyze this question in the following text through the detailed anatomy of metaphors.

Now that we have gone through the main semantic themes of "illness" corpora, let us take a look at the frequent semantic themes of the collocates for "disease" in Table 2-2.

Table 2-2 Main semantic themes of the collocation of "disease"

No.	Item	O1	%1	O2	%2	LL	%DIFF	Semantic Themes
1	B2 −	2099	7.29	1275	0.13 +	10480.10	5.79	Disease
2	B3	599	2.08	1711	0.18 +	1702.33	3.56	Medicines & medical treatment
3	B1	665	2.31	5489	0.57 +	821.10	2.03	Anatomy and physiology
4	B2	90	0.31	129	0.01 +	348.94	4.55	Health and disease
5	A15 −	105	0.36	370	0.04 +	264.19	3.25	Danger
6	X2.4	210	0.73	2176	0.22 +	194.55	1.70	Investigate, examine, test, search
7	A2.2	322	1.12	4362	0.45 +	192.75	1.31	Cause & Effect/Connection
8	S8 −	118	0.41	885	0.09 +	161.77	2.16	Hindering
9	Y1	109	0.38	778	0.08 +	157.23	2.24	Science and technology in general
10	S2	216	0.75	2896	0.30 +	131.84	1.33	People
11	O1	88	0.31	689	0.07 +	115.23	2.10	Substances and materials generally
12	P1	212	0.74	3691	0.38 +	71.86	0.95	Education in general
13	T1.3 +	71	0.25	733	0.08 +	66.12	1.70	Time period: long
14	X2	20	0.07	46	0.00 +	63.50	3.87	Mental actions and processes
15	L2	164	0.57	3225	0.33 +	38.37	0.77	Living creatures: animals, birds
16	W5	29	0.10	225	0.02 +	38.35	2.12	Green issues
17	X5.1 +	34	0.12	344	0.04 +	32.56	1.73	Attentive
18	A2.1 +	179	0.62	3939	0.41 +	27.11	0.61	Change
19	F4	51	0.18	912	0.09 +	16.04	0.91	Farming & Horticulture
20	A1.1.2	44	0.15	815	0.08 +	12.48	0.86	Damaging and destroying

St. 10 Women who attended religious services more than once a week had a 27% lower risk of death from cardiovascular **disease** and a 21% lower **risk of death** from cancer compared with women who never attended.

St. 11 **Risk factors** of coronary artery **disease** in different regions of Saudi Arabia.

As a semantic theme, "Danger" ranked much higher in the collocates of "disease" than it did among the collocates of "illness", which provides more evidence that "disease" is generally perceived as more severe than "illness". Another difference in the meaning between "disease" and "illness" we have mentioned above is that "disease" is usually more concerned with different human organs, while "illness" refers to the general medical problem of human being, especially mental conditions. This argument is also supported with the high-ranking of "Anatomy and physiology" as a semantic theme for "disease". Meanwhile, the theme that is related to "Mental actions and processes" ranked much lower than it did among all the semantic themes of "illness". Example sentences from the theme "Anatomy and physiology" are shown as follows:

- **Anatomy and physiology**

St. 12 We will achieve this through our pioneering research, our vital prevention activity and by ensuring quality care and support for people living with **heart** disease.

St. 13 Long-term use of proton pump inhibitors increases the risk of **kidney** disease.

St. 14 Asthma is a serious chronic disease of the **lungs** that is caused by swelling in the airways.

Apart from its close association with specific human organs, "disease" is also featured by its highlight on infectiousness, especially if the medical problems are caused by the transmission of bacteria or virus from other living creatures to mankind. This argument also finds evidence in the semantic theme "Living creatures" of "disease". This theme is not found in the collocates of "illness", proving that only "disease" is suitable for expressing the medical issues of other living creatures, and it is a better option in describing the medical problems that spread between animals and human beings. Example sentences under this semantic theme include:

- **Living creatures: animals, birds**

St. 15 How it interrelates with its human source of food and with the **parasite** in the maintenance of this devastating **disease**.

St. 16 **Domestic animals** should be inspected for signs of Q fever if people exposed to them have developed symptoms of the **disease**.

St. 17 The **disease** is carried by a tiny **insect** known by various names, including the spittle bug.

St. 18 Butterflies love its orange-red clusters of flowers and it is resistant to **pests** and **diseases**.

In addition, "disease" is more of a professional term used in the medical science and technology than "illness". The fact that semantic themes like "Investigate, examine, test, search", as well as the themes like "Education in general" ranked higher among the themes for "disease" supports our previous argument that "disease" is a more objective, neutral word often used in the field of medical science. For example,

- **Investigate, examine, test, search**

St. 19 We **investigated** the ocular manifestations of this disease in a group of patients drawn from five inflammatory eye **disease** clinics across the United States.

St. 20 In the last few years, through my **research**, I have come to the conclusion, that this increase in **disease**, is caused by our environment.

St. 21 Regulating Prostitution in Late Colonial Bombay, **examines** the moral panics and racialized logics that surrounded 19th- and early 20th-century campaigns to curb brothels, sexually transmitted **disease** and trafficking.

- **Education in general**

St. 22 Although the **study** has pointed out a downside of aspirin, other surveys in recent years have shown protective effects of treatment against various **diseases**.

St. 23 **Follow-up studies** show that breast cancer is a devastating **disease**, with an annual death rate of around 8% among survivors even 20 years after diagnosis.

- **Attentive**

St. 24 The Disease Drivers of Aging: 2016 Advances in Geroscience Summit, held at the New York Academy of Sciences in April 2016, **focused on** three chronic **diseases**: cancer, HIV/AIDS, and diabetes.

St. 25 Overall, the lack of **disease** in the patients with predictive variants **highlights** a lack of understanding of penetrance whether a genetic variant will manifest in disease in an individual, stress Vassy and Rehm.

The above three semantic themes of "disease" all highlight the strong association between "disease" and medical science. The relatively high ranking of the above three themes supports the argument that many words that co-occur with "disease" belong to the reservoir of academic vocabulary. Words like "investigate", "study", "focus on", and "highlight" indicate a strong academic style. The fact that those words often co-occur with "disease" provides further evidence to the objective and professional nature of "disease". Another distinguished feature of "disease" is that the theme "Hindering" enjoys a higher status in all the semantic themes of "disease", as shown in the following examples.

- **Hindering**

St. 26   Exercise not only helps **fight heart disease** by improving all the risk factors, but for sedentary people adding exercise to your daily routine reduces the risk of high blood pressure, osteoporosis, breast and colon cancer, depression, anxiety and stress.

St. 27   We have received letters of appreciation from health workers and families in scores of different countries, often with stories of how they used the book to treat the sick, save lives, and take collective action to **prevent disease**.

St. 28   A diet rich imprint various tocopherol forms may also help to **hinder Alzheimer's disease.**

We can see from the above example sentences that there is an underlying conceptual metaphor behind the "Hindering" theme, which is the war metaphor. The usage of verbs like "fight", "prevent" and "hinder" all implicate that "disease" is visualized as the "marching enemy" toward our "territory", and the only way to "safeguard" our health is through "fighting" with the "disease", so as to "prevent" the "disease" from "attacking" or "harming" our body. War metaphor is one of the most commonly used metaphor when it comes to "disease", and we can learn from the fact that "Hindering" is a more frequent theme in "disease" than in "illness", proving the severity of "disease". Besides, it also sends the message that "disease" is often viewed through a static perspective, when one focuses on characterizing and describing its syndromes, which makes it easier to objectify "disease" and highlight its spacial features. On the contrary, "illness" is usually seen as a dynamic process people go through, emphasizing the unluckiness and dislike towards this annoying period of time.

Thus compared with "disease", "illness" is a more abstract concept measured mainly in the temporal dimension, which makes it a bit harder to visualize "illness" as the enemy we need to fight with.

However, although "illness" is usually perceived as a temporal concept, we do not analyze the phases or stages in the "illness" process. We just see "illness" as a whole process filled with agony and suffering. As to the detailed features of "illness", it is not the main semantic concern. To the opposite, for the word "disease", it is all about looking into, analyzing and studying. Thus, even though "disease" tends to be viewed as a static object with spatial traits, its characteristics in various stages of disease development are also studied. For example, under the theme "Change", the process of disease formation is demonstrated.

- **Change**

St. 29 It has also been found that fish oil reduces the amount of protein in the urine of people who have **developed kidney disease** due to diabetes.

St. 30 Yong Poovorawan, a medical professor at Chulalongkorn University in Bangkok, said an H5N1 strain in the central part of Thailand had **become** resistant to amantadine, casting more doubt over its use to fight the **disease**.

Another interesting distinguished semantic theme of "disease" is "Green issue", which emphasizes the relationship between "disease" and "environment", paying attention to the critical role played by "environmental factors" in the development of diseases. "Green issue" is not found among the semantic theme of "illness". Together with the theme of "Living creatures", "Green issue" also enhances the fact that "disease" is usually the medical problem people contracted from the surroundings, while "illness" is mainly about the state of being ill, especially the mental illness that grows within an individual. Example sentences within the theme of "Green issue" are listed as follows,

St. 31 Study protocol for a randomized controlled trial inflammatory bowel **disease** (IBD) is a chronic condition characterized by recurrent episodes of intestinal inflammation and is thought to be related to an autoimmune reaction to genetic and **environmental factor**.

St. 32 Poorly managed, large scale aquaculture in some countries has **polluted** bays with the accumulation of fish feces and led to escapes of farm-raised stock, threatening wild fish and **spreading disease**.

In summary, after comparing the semantic themes of "disease" and "illness", we have a clearer understanding of the semantic associations of these two words. In general, we can find that the top 3 themes that are relatively overused include "Anatomy and physiology", "Investigate, examine, test and search", and "Science and technology in general", which is consistent with our above analysis. That is, "disease" is more closely related to medical science than to daily conversation about the healthy state of people. However, what's interesting is the following theme—"Farming & Horticulture", which is at first sight irrelevant to the meaning of "disease". The fact that they ranked relatively high in the semantic themes of "disease" suggests the use of metaphors. Thus, we have further analyzed the collocations of "diseases" under the theme "Farming & Horticulture", with an intention to reveal some underlying metaphors in "disease" description in English. First, let us take a look at the word lists within "Farming & Horticulture" theme that collocate with "disease" in the following table.

It can be seen from Table 2-3 that "field" is the most frequent collocate of "disease". It is mainly the frequent usage of "field" when we discuss the researches of various kinds of diseases that contributes to the high-ranking of "Farming & Horticulture" among the semantic themes of "disease", as shown in the following St. 33. Apart from "field", another word that relates the talk about "disease" to the "Farming & Horticulture" is the common use of "breed" in medical science, as shown in St. 34.

Table 2-3 Word list of disease's collocates within "Farming & Horticulture" theme

Rank	Word	Semtag	Frequency	Relative Frequency
1	field	F4	15	0.05
2	breed	F4	4	0.01
3	farmers	F4	4	0.01
4	crops	F4	4	0.01
5	farm	F4	2	0.01

St. 33 To address the **field** diagnosis and control of livestock from this deadly **disease**, the Enzyme Linked Immunosorbent Assay (ELISA) platform was developed in the early 1980s mainly through IAEA support.

St. 34 Members shall never **breed** a Ragdoll whose health or condition show any sign of **disease**, whose temperament is proven faulty due to genetics not environment and/or a Ragdoll which possesses any serious conformation or genetic faults.

Although not evident, we can capture the similarity between doing scientific research and farming, both of which require hard work and aim for "fruitful" results. Moreover, the different disciplines and directions of researches are also frequently expressed by using "Farming & Horticultural" metaphors. Words like "field", "breed" fall into this category. The fact that collocates of "disease" have the "Farming & Horticulture" theme as one of the more common themes again echoes the analysis that discussion of "disease" takes a more objective scientific perspective.

2.1.2 Comparison of the Metaphorical Themes in the Reports on Covid-19 Prevention in China Between *China Daily* and *BBC News*

To identify the potential relevant illness metaphors against the Covid-19 pandemic, we followed the MIP (Metaphor Identification Procedure) of the Pragglejaz Group. The research procedure can be divided into two main parts: First, the manual identification of the metaphorical words in the chosen sample following MIP, and the analysis of the main semantic themes of the sample material using Wmatrix. Second, use the identified metaphorical words as keywords to search for collocates in larger online corpus, analyze the semantic themes of the copora using Wmatrix to see if the semantic themes coincide with the initial analysis of the sample material. The second part of the research provides a quantitative verification of metaphor and semantic theme identification in the first part.

The sample material is chosen from BBC News and *China Daily*. Both articles are concerned with the prevention of Covid-19. The detailed information of the texts are shown as follows:

- Text 1

Name: New Dawn Breaks in Battle Against COVID-19

Source: *China Daily*

Mode: written

Genre, register: newspaper article

Date of composition (or publishing or modification): 2 Dec., 2022

Length of text: 1,478 words

- Text 2

Name: China Covid: New Year Optimism Sees Hopes of Moving Beyond Virus

Source: BBC News

Mode: written

Genre, register: newspaper article

Date of composition (or publishing or modification): 12 Jan., 2023

Length of text: 1,249 words

Guided by the metaphor identifying approaches of MIP, we have asked three doctors in linguistics to code the two texts. To guarantee a strong inter-coder reliability, metaphors with controversy were excluded. Only metaphors that are unanimously agreed by the three coders are listed in the following tables. The identified metaphors are grouped according to the semantic themes they highlight.

Table 2-4 Semantic themes of metaphors in the reports on Covid from *China Daily*

Semantic Fields	Metaphor Words in *China Daily*	Hits
Spatial-temporal	higher (2), peak (1), top (1), stage (1), point (1), gaps (1), adhere to (1), raise (1), overstretched (1), expanded (1), narrowing (2), under pressure (1), downgraded (1), fall (2), center on (1), place (1)	22
Journey/Race	run (1), move (1), stride (1), trajectory (1), overcoming (1), approach (1), direction (1), emerged (3), uneven (2), access (1), entered (1), disrupted (1), step up (2), triumphing (1)	18
War/Violence	battle/fight (4), against (4), hit (2), face (2), stamp out (1), cut (1), targeted (1)	16

(continuous)

Semantic Fields	Metaphor Words in *China Daily*	Hits
Mechanical/Engineering	powerhouse (1), oversimplified (1), one-size-fits-all (1), shortage (1), key (2), tension (1), switched (1), shift (1), linked (1)	10
Explosion	triggered (2), outbreaks (6)	8
Natural disaster / Floods	waves (3), stabilize (1), swept (1), eased (1), riding out (1)	7
Darkness	dawn (3), day breaks in (1), darkness (1), bright (1)	6
Maths/Economics	surge (1), increase (1), rise (1), declined/dropped (2)	5
Person/Human	head (4)	4
House/Container	shielding (1), window (1), containment (1)	3
Process	end/ending (2), phase (1)	3
Total		102

Table 2-5 Semantic themes of metaphors in the reports on Covid from BBC News

Semantic Fields	Metaphor Words in BBC News	Frequency
Math/Economics	had been rising (1), surge (6), rebound (2), decline/drop (6), caseload (1), soar (1)	17
Spatial-temporal	trending downward (1), raise (1), down (2), over (2), narrowing (1), underreported (1), low (1), spike (1), around (1), fully (1), peak (2)	14
Person	position (1), eyes/see (2), bittersweet (1), experiencing (3), head (1), appearing (1), struggling (1), cope with (1)	11
Dominance	track down variants (1), lifted (6), relaxed/eased (2), curbs (1)	10
Natural disaster / Floods	wave / the first huge wave / a large Covid wave (9)	9
Process	coming to an end / timing of an end / ended (5)	5
War/Violence	against (3), hit (1)	4
Journey/Race	run (1), beyond Covid (1), Covid losses mount (1)	3
Explosion	trigger (2), explosion of cases (1)	3
Behemoth Monster	in the grip of (1), the virus tore (1)	2
Mechanic/Engineering	linked to Covid (2)	2
Total		80

Chapter 2 Corpus-Based Comparison of Disease Metaphors in English and Chinese

The above Table 2-5 displays the main semantic themes of metaphors identified in the article on Covid-19 in BBC news. By comparing the above two tables, we can find that in general the article from *China Daily* has more metaphorical expressions than the report in BBC News. The number of words in the texts from *China Daily* and BBC News is similar, yet the article from *China Daily* has 102 metaphorical expressions, while the article from BBC News on the same topic (Covid) has only 80 metaphorical expressions, much less than that of *China Daily*.

The main differences between the above two tables lie in the ranking of the following semantic themes: "War/Violence", "Dominance", and "Math/Economics". Now let us take a further look at the specific metaphors used in the above three themes from *China Daily* and BBC News. First, War/Violence (16) ranks very high in the semantic themes from the text of *China Daily*, while there are only 4 hits in War/Violence from the text of BBC News.

St. 1   In the second quarter of this year, the protracted **fight** against the disease as it swept across the economic powerhouse of Shanghai raised concerns over sustainability of the strategy.

St. 2   For most of this year, China adhered to its dynamic zero-COVID-19 policy, which called for prompt and precise control measures to **stamp out** domestic outbreaks.

St. 3   February, the highly transmissible Omicron strain of the virus triggered frequent and widespread outbreaks, "posing the most severe test since the initial outbreak **hit** Wuhan, Hubei Province, the hardest".

In the above example sentences, although Covid-19 is viewed as a strong enemy, China is more perceived as a persistent and capable fighter, who insists on fighting against the enemy and can withstand the attack from Covid. The adoption of "War/Violence" metaphor actually posits China in a strong position against the virus, which demonstrates a positive attitude in the fight against the enemy. The verbs like "fight / hit / stamp out" are all of strong agency, laying more emphasis on China's pro-activity. When the focus is more concentrated on China's initiative and power, the threat of the virus is relatively downplayed.

Different from the highlight on China's pro-activity using "War/Violence" metaphor, in terms of the relationship between China and Covid-19, the correspondent main semantic theme adopted in BBC News is viewing China more as a person who is affected by the virus. In this case, the semantic theme that ranks high in BBC News is "Person". For example,

Title: China **Eyes** Life Beyond Covid Despite High Infections.

St. 4 The country is **seeing** a surge in cases since the lifting of its most severe restrictions earlier this month.

St. 5 China has been **experiencing** a surge in Covid cases since many restrictions were eased earlier this month.

It can be seen from the above examples that China is more viewed as a common human being rather than a competent power against the enemy. The relationship between China and Covid is not perceived as a war, of which both the two sides can take initiatives, and the side that is stronger and more competent stands a higher chance of winning the battle. Rather, China is seen as a person who is passively undergoing the suffering and hardship caused by Covid-19. The verbs like "see and experience" are low in agency, which can not demonstrate one's proactivity. If we say that in the article of *China Daily*, China is more perceived as a "fighter", while in the news from BBC, China is seen as a "person". The fact of BBC News employs more metaphors of the "Person" theme also reflects its intention to downplay the efforts made by the Chinese government in preventing the virus and protecting the lives of Chinese citizens. Especially when the Western government is not playing a more active role in handling the disease, which resulted in a large number of deaths among their citizens, Western media like BBC are unwilling to report the persistent efforts Chinese government have made in curbing the pandemic. In addition, in the article of *China Daily*, "Person" metaphor is restricted to the word "head", which is used to refer to the "leaders" of organizations.

Although BBC News adopts more "Person" metaphors in the reports of China's handling of Covid-19, ironically, the then Prime Minister of the UK, Boris Johnson resorted to "War" metaphor when he was addressing the British Media. On the 17th March 2020, 5 days before the United Kingdom was put under lockdown due to the Covid-19 pandemic, Boris Johnson made an official statement that included the following:

Chapter 2 Corpus-Based Comparison of Disease Metaphors in English and Chinese

Yes this **enemy** can be deadly, but it is also **beatable**, and we know how to **beat it and we know that if as a country** we follow the scientific advice that is now being given we know that we will **beat** it.

And however tough the **months ahead** we have the resolve and the resources to win the **fight**.

We can see from the speech made by Boris Johnson that he is clearly using "War" metaphor to depict the current scenario. Words like "enemy", "beatable", "beat", and "fight" all contribute to the narrative that the British people were facing a "war" against the corona virus. Naturally, in the middle of a war, unity of the country is further stressed. Resolution is what the "country" needs to "win the fight". Besides, in his speech, a long-term dynamic perspective is employed, which can be reflected in the phrase "months ahead", asking the British citizens to go through the "tough" period together and laying stress on the future prospect.

Interestingly, the metaphors and perspectives applied in the above speech is very much the same with those used in *China Daily*, while quite the opposite to the metaphors used in BBC's report on China's Covid-19 prevention measures. The evident change of tone reveals the double standards of BBC News. When the British government attempts to appeal to British people's emotion to boost confidence in overcoming the disease and to cooperate with the lockdown measures, they deem that as necessary approaches needed in the special period of time. However, when the exact same measures were taken by Chinese government, it is viewed by BBC News as an ill-intended way to dominate and manipulate the people against their free will. The subconscious bias and embedded stereotype against a country with different political system is clouding the judgement of BBC News and some other Western media in a way that they do not even realize.

Apart from the different semantic themes employed by *China Daily* and BBC News in terms of the relationship between China and Covid-19, the texts selected from these two sources also demonstrate a clear contrast in the perception of the measures taken in pandemic prevention. In *China Daily*, "Journey/Race" semantic theme ranked as the second most frequent theme when it comes to Covid prevention, words like "run" (1), "move" (1), "stride" (1), "trajectory" (1), "overcoming" (1), "approach" (1), "direction" (1), "emerged" (3), "uneven" (2), "access" (1), "entered" (1), "disrupted" (1), "step up" (2), "triumphing" (1) all indicate the visualization of the whole fight of Covid as a journey or a race. When Covid-19 prevention is seen as a "journey", we assume there is a destination or end to it, thus what needs to be done is to persist and keep going. Similarly, when Covid-19 prevention is perceived as a "race", thus one needs faster speed and stamina to succeed. Example sentences are listed as follows.

St. 6 While abiding by the dynamic zero-COVID policy, we are also upgrading virus control measures and seizing the window of opportunity created by the policy to **step up** preparedness for ultimately **triumphing** over the disease.

St. 7 The second wave will be triggered by increased movement during the Spring Festival from late January to mid-February, while the third, from late February to mid-March, will be linked to migrant employees returning to their workplaces, Wu said during a speech titled "How to **Stride** Over the Darkness Before the Dawn".

St. 8 "The three waves constitute the **trajectory** of this winter's epidemic. By overcoming this winter season, we will see a bright spring," he said.

The above examples demonstrate the holistic view towards Covid-29 prevention in the articles from *China Daily*. Words like "step up", "triumphing", "stride over" as well as "trajectory" are all viewing Covid-29 either as a journey or a race, both of which have a destination or a goal. Psychologically, setting goal or destination can boost the motivation of people, so those who are experiencing the inconvenience caused by Covid-19 prevention measures are more willing to endure the temporary hardship. Another assumption under the "Journey/Race" metaphor is that it puts everyone in the same path, and there is one way out for everyone. So all we need to do and have to do is to keep on going forward, since persistence is the right direction for both the government and people. This can also endow the country and people with more enduring power and collective strength to go through the hard time together.

Another clear contrast in the frequency of semantic themes between *China Daily* and BBC News resides in the use of metaphors from "Math/Economics" field. It can be seen from Tables 2-4 and 2-5 that there are 17 hits under "Math/Economics" theme, which ranks the first among all the semantic themes adopted in the article, while there are only 5 records in "Math/Economics" theme for the article selected from *China Daily*. As shown in the text details, the articles from two sources are published during the similar time span, around the end of 2022 and the beginning of 2023. And the articles are all reports on the Covid situation in China. The similarity in time and topic provides us with the common ground for comparison and contrast.

At the end of 2022, China's Covid prevention measure is going through a series of shifts and changes. From the article of BBC News, many metaphorical expressions frequently used in "Math/Economics" field are used to stress the change in the number. Words like "rising" (1), "surge" (6), "rebound" (2), "decline/drop" (6), "caseload" (1), "soar" (1) are common in the reports, which can create a sense that the arguments are evidence-based and supported with statistical evidence. For example,

St. 9 Fears that the virus could **surge** again during the festive period have also not yet been realised.

St. 10 "We will know soon if the Lunar New Year celebrations will trigger another **surge** in China cases, but it is unlikely to match what was experienced in December and the earlier part of January 2023."

St. 11 Meanwhile, China's largest city, Shanghai, has ordered most of its schools to take classes online as cases **soar**.

St. 12 But experts say the **decline** reported now corresponds with the expected timing of an end to this major wave.

It can be seen from the above examples that the report on China's dealing with Covid from BBC News in-proportionately highlights the possible increase of the number of cases and Covid death. Verbs like "surge", "soar", "rise" are the frequent choice when it comes to the number. Despite the fact that numbers themselves are neutral, the stress on the sudden change of cases intends to make people feel anxious about the change, which also insinuates a sense of uncertainty about the future, increasing the unsecured feeling and enhancing a pessimistic view on what is going to happen after. The choice of the verbs like "surge and soar" also highlights the instability and enlarges one's fear about the uncertain future.

Thus the seemingly objective and neutral statistics were also selected and presented based on one's attitude and position. Those "Math/Economics" words are not purely statistical after all, on the contrary, they help to frame the situation as a kind of "crisis", which enlarges the negative impression of the current situation. Meanwhile, the article from *China Daily* does not apply many metaphors from the "Math/Economics" theme, but the article does introduce the situation using more "Spatial-temporal" metaphors. For example,

St. 13   He said those joining the holiday travel rush face a **higher** risk of infection and they should continue to take precautions against the virus and practice personal protection.

St. 14   "We are certainly in a much better **place** with the pandemic than a year ago, when we were in the early stages of the Omicron wave with rapidly increasing cases and deaths," he said. "Since the **peak** at the end of January, the number of COVID-19 deaths reported weekly has dropped by almost 90 percent."

St. 15   He said detecting new infections quickly, **expanding** the capacity of quarantine facilities, designated and makeshift hospitals, and formulating targeted treatment protocols for COVID-19 patients experiencing the disease with different levels of severity were key to the strategy during this period.

St. 16   Wang Guangfa, head of Peking University First Hospital's respiratory illness and critical care department, said hospitals are **under pressure** to handle a large number of fever cases, people requesting emergency care due to cold weather, and patients with chronic diseases that have been worsened by COVID-19.

St. 17   In the second quarter of this year, the protracted fight against the disease as it swept across the economic powerhouse of Shanghai **raised** concerns over sustainability of the strategy.

St. 18   If we abandon virus control measures altogether, our healthcare system will be **overstretched**, lives of vulnerable groups will be threatened, and the overall development of society and the economy will be disrupted.

From the above examples, we can see the situation in China from a different angle. Instead of stressing the "suddenness" of change in the number of cases, which will cause more panic and fear among the public, the article from *China*

Chapter 2　Corpus-Based Comparison of Disease Metaphors in English and Chinese

Daily is adopting a holistic and dynamic perspective in discussing the matters related to the increase of cases and the pressure of the medical system. Rather than using "verbs" which might add to the sense of uneasiness, more "nouns" and "adjectives" are used to describe the rationality of the situation in a calmer manner. For example, compared with "the number of case is surging", "a higher risk" is much less frightening. "A higher risk" is a more objective and scientific evaluation of the situation, acknowledging the risk while giving readers assurance of "under control". Besides, reasons for the "higher risk" is also provided in the sentence, which is "the holiday travel rush". Compared with "rising", "raised" has a clear subject, which allows people to see the whole picture, the reasons and whereabouts. A complete rational logical analysis can ease one's anxiety, cause people to become anxious in a clueless situation. However, as we have analyzed in the article from BBC News, attention is paid solely to the action, without explaining the reasons and results.

Similarly, the word "peak" sends out two messages: The first is that the current number of cases was big, and the second is that it was going to drop after, of which the second message is louder than the first one, thus providing more comfort to the public. And the holistic view across the long-time span also reduced people's anxiety at the moment. Apart from the choice of words, the focus in sentences of the article of *China Daily* is on "problem-solving", words like "under pressure" and "overstretched" are emphasizing the possible difficulties in hospital. The message delivered is that the government and the hospitals are doing their best to save more lives despite the increased number of infections. However, the mere presentation of statistical changes in BBC News is more about "the severity of the problem", creating an impression that the problem will cause many damages while ignoring the fact that efforts can be made to deal with the problem.

In addition, another theme that only appears in the report of Covid-19 in *China Daily* is "Housing" theme, including words like "shield", "contain", "window". Example sentences are:

St. 19　The nation has switched from prompt and precise **containment** of domestic outbreaks of the disease to **shielding** the most vulnerable groups and dedicating all-out efforts to treating patients in serious condition.

Cognitive and Contrastive Analysis of Disease Metaphors in English and Chinese

St. 20 "While abiding by the dynamic zero-COVID policy, we are also upgrading virus control measures and seizing the **window** of opportunity created by the policy to step up preparedness for ultimately triumphing over the disease."

In the above examples, the pandemic is seen as the spreading evil that needs to be "contained". The Chinese government was trying their very best to "contain" the virus and "shield" people from the infection, especially the vulnerable groups like the senior citizens and patients in serious condition. The "House/Container" metaphor is not found in the article from BBC News. For *China Daily*, the activation of the "Housing" theme can also serve to sooth the nerves of the public, and make people less worried about the situation. Besides, by stressing government's role in providing "shield" to people in difficult times, and highlighting the efforts made to "contain" the evil virus, the faith of people in the government can be enhanced.

The comparison between the BBC's frequent usage of "Math/Economics" theme and *China Daily*'s emphasis on "Spatial-temporal" metaphors reveals the position of both sides. In general, BBC's report on China's Covid situation attempts to play the role of an objective third-party evaluator by presenting "statistical facts". However, the way the numbers are presented, the choice of verbs, and the information that it withholds, all contribute to "bend" the reality in the way they want. Meanwhile, *China Daily* describes the situation from their perspectives, which stresses the holistic and dynamic picture of the long fight against Covid, and the government's efforts made to face up to the challenges. By doing so, Chinese government was providing more confidence to the public in overcoming the hardship, and persuading people to have faith in the government and in themselves. As the old saying in Chinese puts, "While prospects are bright, the roads have twists and turns." A distinctive "theme" applied in the article from *China Daily* is "Darkness", which is consistent with the above analysis. "Darkness" metaphor is employed specifically to enhance people's faith in the ultimate success against the virus. Typical metaphors included under this theme include the following examples:

Title: New **Dawn** Breaks in Battle Against COVID-19

St. 21 The shift of focus in China's COVID-19 containment strategy signals a

Chapter 2 Corpus-Based Comparison of Disease Metaphors in English and Chinese

new dawn in the battle against the virus, according to officials and experts.

St. 22   The second wave will be triggered by increased movement during the Spring Festival from late January to mid-February, while the third, from late February to mid-March, will be linked to migrant employees returning to their workplaces, Wu said during a speech titled "How to Stride Over the **Darkness Before the Dawn**".

St. 23   "The three waves constitute the trajectory of this winter's epidemic. By overcoming this winter season, we will see a **bright spring**," he said.

It can be seen from the above examples that the current hardship is placed in a wider and longer spatial-temporal dimension. The emphasis on the "brightness" of "dawn" and the "warmth" of "spring" can reduce the spreading of pessimism and boosts people's confidence in overcoming the disease. Given that the phrase "darkness before the dawn" was originally used to describe the darkest moment before winning a war, the usage of "dawn" metaphor in describing activities in fighting Covid-19 is also alluding to the fact that there is a war between human and the virus. And the war has come to a critical moment, what takes to win the battle is a bit more persistence. The narrative can indeed unite people together during the hard time and strengthen people's determination in defeating the coronavirus and getting their lives back on the normal track.

Now that we have discussed the differences in the semantic themes of reports on Covid in China from BBC News and *China Daily*, there are also some similarities in the used metaphors between the two sources. Both sides possess a relatively large number of metaphors within "Spatial-temporal" theme and "Natural disasters". Based on the common cognitive rules of human beings, "Spatial-temporal" metaphors are the most fundamental conceptual metaphors in our conceptualization of the world. Thus it is not surprising that "Spatial-temporal" metaphors are common in the reports of both. Besides, "Natural disaster", especially "floods", is also a common original domain in many cultures, and it frequently projected onto other phenomena that bring huge damage or harm to human civilization.

In the articles of *China Daily* and BBC News, the infection Covid-19 cases are compared to "wave". Metaphors of this theme are used 9 times in the report on

53

China's Covid situation and 7 metaphorical expressions within the "Floods" theme can be identified in the article from *China Daily*. For example,

St. 24 Wu Zunyou, chief epidemiologist at the Chinese Center for Disease Control and Prevention, said the country will be hit by three **waves** of COVID-19 this winter, with the first centering on urban areas until the middle of next month. (*China Daily*)

St. 25 Experts said the key to **riding out the wave** of infections is to reduce the scale of outbreaks to below the full capacity level of medical systems and increase protection for vulnerable members of society. (*China Daily*)

St. 26 Chinese health officials say the country's current **wave** of Covid-19 infections is "coming to an end". (BBC News)

St. 27 But experts say the decline reported now corresponds with the expected timing of an end to this major **wave**. (BBC News)

As shown above, both *China Daily* and BBC News used "Waves" to depict the infection. However, the active players in the sentence are different. In St. 26 and 27, "current wave" or "major wave" is the only active player in the scenario, establishing a situation where the Covid "wave" has already or about to dominate the country, the omission of measures taken by human beings leaves "wave" the only pivotal role, creating a rather pessimistic view of the situation. On the other hand, although the same "Floods" theme is activated in the article from *China Daily*. The metaphorical word "wave" is depicted as an intruder in the country. China is the main subject of the sentence. In St. 24, passive voice is used to stress the "intrusion" of the Covid-19 "wave". Yet China is seen as an active player in the battle, which can withstand the "hit" and still erect in the whole scenario. Similarly, in St. 25, China has a more active interaction with the "wave", and the focus is on China's active planning to "ride out" safely in the Covid infection wave. Still, the theme under "Natural disasters" in Chinese narrative always pays tribute to man's will and power. That is, regardless of the destroying power of "Floods" or other "Natural disasters", man can always survive, defend their territory and claim the final triumph. Whereas the article from BBC News tends to tell a different story, downplaying the man power and highlighting the invincibility of "Natural disasters".

Chapter 2 Corpus-Based Comparison of Disease Metaphors in English and Chinese

As to philosophy concerning the relationship between man and Nature, traditional Chinese philosophy emphasizes the harmony between the two, arguing that man should abide by the law of Nature and carry out human activities according to the natural tendency. There seems to exist a contradictory understanding towards the human nature relationship. However, if one looks further into Chinese people's life philosophy, one would find the seemingly contradictory understandings actually are united under the keyword, that is, the "balance" between man and Nature. What underlines the harmonious relationship between man and Nature is the power balance between the two. Since "keeping balance" is the key, thus the side that breaks the balance will be punished, and eventually the balance will be restored. Guided by this philosophy, the Chinese people are more resilient during the hardship of Covid infection, because deep down they believe that the "tide" rise and fall, the "waves" come and go, balance will be restored one way or another.

It is a sense of equity behind the balance philosophy. Man is not seen as powerful as Nature. Instead, man is expected to view Nature power with awe. But at the same time, man's power is not dwindled or dwarfed by the magnificent natural force, instead, human being is placed on the equal status with Nature. Therefore, when humans are enduring the "roar" and "fury" of Nature, we are entitled to "fight" for our own survival, and stand a chance of "riding out" the "wave" with our will, strength and persistence.

This man and Nature philosophy is echoed by the use of metaphors in "Mechanic/Engineering" theme, which is a vivid display of manpower in the industrialized age. "Mechanic/Engineering" is the fourth most frequent semantic theme in the report from *China Daily*, which is in clear contrast to its records in BBC News. Only two "hits" are documented of metaphorical expressions under this theme of the article from BBC News. The metaphorical words used under this theme are "powerhouse" (1), "oversimplified" (1), "one-size-fits-all" (1), "shortage" (1), "key" (2), "tension" (1), "switched" (1), "shift" (1), "linked" (1). Example sentences are as follows.

St. 28 The nation has **switched** from prompt and precise containment of domestic outbreaks of the disease to shielding the most vulnerable groups and dedicating all-out efforts to treating patients in serious condition.

St. 29　By July, 12 government departments and authorities in all 31 provincial-level regions had set up channels to gather complaints about **oversimplified** disease control measures, the adoption of a "**one-size-fits-all approach**", or the enforcement of additional restrictions, the commission said.

St. 30　Infections among healthcare staff members have also increased **tension**.

We can see from the above example sentences that the source domains of words like "switch", "one-size-fits-all approach" are "Mechanic/Engineering", which is the result of human industrialized civilization. By using the words and phrases within the genre of science and technology, the Covid prevention activities can also be seen as planned and organized based on scientific methods. Besides, discussing the "virus" in scientific language also enhances the narrative that the situation is under control and can be dealt with. In other words, using "Mechanic/Engineering" theme to describe the Covid pandemic can reduce the uncertainty about its development, for the "Mechanic/Engineering" theme symbolizes order and structure, which reduces randomness and chaotic feeling. The fact that very few metaphors within this theme are identified in the report from BBC News indicates that the Western media chose the language style they deemed suitable and framed the information in the way that was in line with their intention.

In summary, the semantic themes of the metaphors used in articles from *China Daily* and BBC News possess both similarities and differences. In terms of similarities, both sides use many "Spatial-temporal" metaphors and "Natural disasters" metaphors, although the specific application in the context differs in the semantic emphasis. The differences exist in the usage of several semantic themes, which can be summarized into the following four main points: (1) *China Daily* depicts the virus as the enemy of the whole country and the mankind, thus using many metaphorical expressions within the "War/Violence" theme, of which China and mankind are seen as the "fighter" against the virus; meanwhile, BBC News sees the virus as the "behemoth monster", highlighting its destroying power against human beings, and views China more as a weak "patient" who is unlikely to withstand the attack of the virus. (2) *China Daily* tended to describe the Covid prevention as a long journey or a race against virus, and Chinese government and the

Chinese people were in the same team. Thus in order to "win" the "race" against the virus, the whole country needed to stay united and not to give in to the virus despite the hardship and inconvenience in the meantime caused by strict prevention measures. (3) *China Daily* adopts a holistic and dynamic view when discussing the changes in number of infections, using more "Spatial-temporal" metaphors to present the situation in a more rational and objective way. To the opposite, BBC News relies more on "Math/Economics" metaphors to stress the instability and highlight the change in numbers only at the moment. By adopting the micro and static perspective, the article from BBC News appealed to the readers' anxiety and fear in the disguise of seemingly neutral numbers and facts. (4) *China Daily* used more metaphors from the "Mechanic/Engineering" theme to place the Covid infection in scientific discourse, which enhanced the objectivity in dealing with the virus, and increased the degree of certainty in prevention activities. However, metaphors from this theme was rarely used in the article from BBC News. Instead, the virus is compared to "behemoth monster" that holds China "in the grip" and may "tear" China apart, which tended to increase the fear and anxiety of the public.

2.2 Distribution of Typical Conceptual Metaphors in the Self-Established Corpus of *China Daily* and BBC News

In this section, attention is paid to the identification and categorization of major metaphorical domains in the established corpus, both the *China Daily* corpus and the corpus based on BBC News. Besides, frequent metaphorical themes devoted specifically to pandemic prevention will also be discussed.

2.2.1 Identification of Frequent Metaphor Words and Key Domains in the Corpus

After comparing the metaphorical themes in the two texts on Covid in China from *China Daily* and BBC News, we were able to locate some frequent metaphor words. Eliminating the functional words, we selected the frequent metaphor words that are content words, that is, words with more specific referents. The words are shown in Table 2-6.

Table 2-6 Frequent metaphorical words and phrases from the two texts on Covid-19

Spatial-temporal	peak, raise, expand, fall, high, down, over, low	+
War	battle, fight, against, hit, face, target	--
Journey	run, step up, entered, direction, move	--
Natural disaster	wave, sweep, ease, ride out	+
Person	eyes, see, experience, head, struggle	++
Explosion	trigger, outbreak	+
Maths	increase, rise, surge, decline, drop, soar	++
House/Container	shield, window, contain	--
Monster	grip, tear	++

In order to further analyze the metaphorical themes used in describing Covid-19 in China, we first collected all the reports on Covid in China from BBC News, which includes 290 articles, and the total number of words is 167,280. Then we used the same keywords "China", "Covid" to search for reports in *China Daily* and collected 320 articles, the total number of words is 172,030. Then we uploaded both txt files to Wmatrix for semantic tagging. After comparing the semantically tagged file from BBC News and the file from *China Daily* with BNC written as the reference corpus, we have identified the top 10 overused semantic themes in both files, as shown in the following figures.

```
                        Corpus Analysis
              The top 10 key domains are: (full list)
List Context B3      1102    Medicines and medical treatment
List Context Z2      3919    Geographical names
List Context B2-     943     Disease
List Context Z99     12208   Unmatched                        Change cut off:
List Context G1.1    1457    Government                       10    Go
List Context T1.3    2165    Time: Period
List Context B2      240     Health and disease
List Context Q2.1    1678    Speech: Communicative
List Context Q4.3    379     The Media: TV, Radio and Cinema
List Context Q4      391     The Media
              The top 10 words in each of these domains are:
 B3 full list vaccines vaccine hospitals medical hospital vaccination vaccinated healthcare medicine treatment
 Z2 full list China chinese Beijing Shanghai Wuhan India UK Hong_Kong var Singapore
 B2- full list pandemic outbreak infections patients disease outbreaks infection symptoms epidemic fever
 Z99 full list covid covid-19 zero-covid lockdown TopicsCoronavirus panelshare pagecopy linkabout https coronavirus
 G1.1full list country government officials authorities official president state citizens ministry congress
 T1.3full list January year days December week months December_2022 years day month
 B2 full list health infected asymptomatic mental_health influenza coughing health_sector diarrhoea endemic cough
 Q2.1full list said told says say content saying statement response state comment
 Q4.3full list video videos Footage tv transmitted broadcaster filmed viewers transmission CCTV
 Q4 full list media published censorship publishing censors title coverage censored censor publish
```

Figure 2-1 Top 10 overused semantic themes in reports on Covid in China from BBC News

Chapter 2 Corpus-Based Comparison of Disease Metaphors in English and Chinese

		Corpus Analysis		
		The top 10 key domains are: (full list)		
List	Context Z2	5531	Geographical names	
List	Context M7	3095	Places	
List	Context Y1	891	Science and technology in general	
List	Context S8+	2043	Helping	Change cut off:
List	Context Z99	6103	Unmatched	10 Go
List	Context I2.2	1426	Business: Selling	
List	Context I2.1	1327	Business: Generally	
List	Context G1.1	1504	Government	
List	Context I4	490	Industry	
List	Context A2.1+	1383	Change	
		The top 10 words in each of these domains are:		
Z2	full list	China chinese Beijing asian Asia United_States Shanghai Taiwan Kenya Africa		
M7	full list	countries international province foreign local region city national areas cities		
Y1	full list	technology science scientific technological technologies high-tech space_station quantum scientists astronauts		
S8+	full list	cooperation support help promote services promoting boost protection service assistance		
Z99	full list	covid-19 — year-on-year china-central photo/xinl 编辑(Alt + A) juancun coercive zhang shanxi //		
I2.2	full list	trade market sales exports trading imports consumer markets agency consumers		
I2.1	full list	economy companies business enterprises infrastructure company businesses ltd economies insurance_companies		
G1.1	full list	country President government bureau state governance revenue authorities official governments		
I4	full list	industrial industry industries data_industry insurance_industry factory mining semiconductor_industry industrialization coal_mining		
A2.1+	full list	development become change transformation developing developed develop reform changes momentum		

Figure 2-2 Top 10 overused semantic themes in reports on Covid in China from *China Daily*

By comparing the above two figures, we can find that both BBC News and *China Daily* have overused the semantic themes like "Geographical names" and "Government". This is easy to be understood since both of the two files are news reports, which would definitely include more words and phrases to answer the "Where" question. And given that one of the searching keywords is "China", so naturally "Government" would be a main theme in the corpus.

However, it is interesting to notice that apart from these two themes, the other 8 overused semantic themes are all different. We can learn from Figure 1 that "Disease", "Medicines and medical treatment", as well as "Health and disease" are overused in BBC's reports on Covid in China. Since the keywords used for searching include "Covid", so it is reasonable that themes related to "Disease", "Medicines and medical treatment", "Health and disease" are overused. However, the overuse of themes related to "Speech" and "Media" is unexpected. When we take a further look at the frequent words included in "Speech" and "Media", we can notice that the stress is laid on the "opinion, comment" rather than the fact, for example, we find words like "said", "told", "saying", "state" frequently used.

Meanwhile, themes like "Science and technology", "Helping" and "Change" are the overused semantic themes in *China Daily*'s reports on Covid in China. Quite to the opposite of the semantic themes used in BBC News, *China Daily*'s reports on Covid in China actually do not overuse themes related to

"Medicine" or "Disease", despite the fact that the collected articles are related to Covid in China. Apart from the mentioning of "Covid" in the unmatched theme, all the other 9 themes are not related to "Disease" at all. Instead, we have themes that are addressing the "Industry", "Science and technology", and "Business". Besides, more positive themes are overused, like "Helping", including frequent words like "cooperation", "support", "promote", and themes that are future-oriented, such as "Change", which is emphasizing the "change" after the pandemic.

Through the comparison of the overused themes in *China Daily* and BBC News, we can sense that in the reports of *China Daily*, the pandemic is over and the country is recovering quickly in all respects. However, BBC's narrative about Covid in China still holds onto the situation before the change of Covid-control policy, which is already outdated.

Another theme that is frequently used in BBC's reports on China's Covid prevention is "Isolation". Compared with the word "quarantine", "isolation" connotes a more negative preference. According to the dictionary definition, "quarantine" refers to "a period of time when an animal or a person that has or may have a disease is kept away from others in order to prevent the disease from spreading", which is more of a professional neutral term commonly used in the scientific field, especially in epidemiology. Meanwhile, the word "isolation" can be used both to professionally mean "separate for medical purpose" and generally refers to the "state of being isolated", which entails a negative emotional value. According to the Word Frequency List, "isolation" used 17 times in BBC's report on the measures taken by China to cope with the spreading virus, while the word "isolation" only appeared 9 times in *China Daily*'s report on China's Covid prevention. Given the similar size and common topic between the two datasets, we can conclude that "isolation" is used more frequently in BBC's report with a semantic preference on its negative pragmatic color, for example.

St. 1 China follows a "zero Covid" strategy, including mass testing, **strict isolation** rules and local lockdowns. This has resulted in far fewer deaths than in many other countries.

St. 2 Officials have also started to transform China's Covid **isolation centres**

Chapter 2 Corpus-Based Comparison of Disease Metaphors in English and Chinese

into temporary hospital facilities, to cope with an explosion of infections.

St. 3 It has had three years to prepare for an eventual reopening, but instead of building more hospital ICU units and emphasizing the need for vaccinations, it has poured enormous resources into mass testing, lockdown and **isolation facilities** designed to win a war against a virus which is never going away.

We can see from the above examples that "isolation" is repeatedly used to highlight the sheer strictness in China's Covid prevention measures. The phrase "isolation center" conveys a sense of distance and indifference, while the fact is that many quarantine centers are rather comfortable, and most of the people who spend a period of time in quarantine center were being taken care of both physically and mentally.

In the reports from *China Daily*, "isolation" is not so frequently used as in BBC News. And in the 9 sentences that do use the word "isolation", the word is not used to refer to the quarantine center, but to describe more abstract concepts, like "political" or "economic" isolation, as shown in the following examples,

St. 4 Facing economic and social problems in the US, then president Barack Obama adopted the Pivot to Asia policy in 2011, targeting China's rise with a containment policy of military expansion and **economic isolation**.

St. 5 From economic sanctions to technical blockade, and from **political isolation** to threat of force, the US has demonstrated what coercive diplomacy is to the world with its own actions.

The fact that BBC News deliberately uses "isolation" to refer to the quarantine center in China reflects their intolerance of Chinese government's different yet effective approach in curbing the spread of coronavirus. Given the difference in political systems, the measures carried out in China may be not suitable for Western countries, but that does not give the Western media like BBC News the rights to "isolate" China. Merely because China is adopting different policies in handling Covid-19 pandemic, many Western media tend to see China as a "heretic". Not only did BBC News backgrounded China's efforts in effectively containing the virus through lockdown, quarantine and virus tracking, it also attempts to deny the measures completely for some inconvenience caused by mismanagement or incapability in some areas.

Apart from the frequent themes related to "Medicines and medical treatment", "Geographical names", "Disease", and "Time:Period", another semantic theme that is not in line with the topic of the material is the "Color/Colorful pattern", which ranks high according to LogDice value among the semantic themes in BBC's report on China's Covid prevention. It seems hard to understand in the first place. After looking into the contexts for words denoting "color", we have found out the reasons. The high frequency of "colorful words" is due to the reports on the "Health Code" system implemented by the Chinese government in order to better track people's movement, so as to cut the transmission of virus as quickly as possible. The repeated usage of "color" words reflect the Western media's intention in politicizing the measures taken to contain the pandemic. The overuse of the word "Red" is the most significant. Red, which is simply the color of the health code, indicates that the person has a higher chance of being affected by coronavirus,

St.6 QR codes are bar codes that can be read by mobile phones. Under the scheme China has employed since February, users are issued a **traffic-light style health code**, with a **green code** allowing someone to travel freely, and **an orange or red code** indicating that they need to quarantine for up to two weeks.

In St.6, the health code system is not aimed to control, but means to protect the citizens. The restrictions and inconvenience caused in the process are the means for the better ends, that is, people's health and lives, especially the health and lives of the vulnerable groups. That is why it is called "health code", being "colorful" is not the point, the point is it can indeed slow down the transmission through in-time information sharing. To some extent, the "health code" system does resemble "traffic lights", only the similarities lie in the fact that both of them aim to protect lives. Even the same metaphor can be interpreted differently depending on one's perspective and underlying assumptions.

Besides the choice of words and the highlight of certain semantic themes, the metaphors used in BBC News and *China Daily* in describing Covid-19 are also different. Among all the common metaphorical themes used in discussing Covid-19 pandemic (Table 2-6), one of the most frequent one is the "War/Violence"

Chapter 2 Corpus-Based Comparison of Disease Metaphors in English and Chinese

metaphors. Using the typical word "fight" as an example, we have found 25 "fight" and 5 "fighting" used in the reports from *China Daily*, while the word "fight" as a verb only appeared less than 13 times, and 3 of them are not directly related to Covid. Even among the remaining 10 sentences that include the metaphorical word "fight", the subjects of the sentence are mostly individuals rather than China as a country or the mankind in general. On the contrary, in the altogether 30 "fight/fighting" identified in the reports from *China Daily*, 29 are directly related to the "fight" against Covid, and the subjects of the sentence are mostly about China, mankind or the globe as a whole, for example,

St. 7   This indicates the **fight between humans and COVID-19** may continue for some time to come.

St. 8   Given the numbers of infections, at around 100,500, and related deaths, at around 4,600, recorded over the past more than two years, and the relatively swift resumption of economic activities, **China's fight against the COVID-19 pandemic** should be considered successful.

St. 9   Perhaps having been prompted by the failure of the advanced countries, especially the US, to fulfil their commitment to the **global fight against the pandemic**, the UNAIDS Executive Director Winnie Byanyima had once commented that "empty promises will not save the world from COVID-19".

St. 10   China has stood out and played a significant role in the **global fight against the COVID-19** pandemic over the past three years, experts and officials said.

It can be seen from the above examples that "War" metaphor is indeed a frequent metaphor used in *China Daily*'s reports on China's handling with Covid-19 pandemic. And the "War" is more perceived as the battle between the whole country, the world, and the mankind against the virus. It is not a "fight" between individuals and the virus, but a "fight" that calls for "unity" among the Chinese people, between different countries, and across continents. From the perspective of China, the whole world should cooperate in defeating the virus to protect lives around the globe.

However, going through the contexts for "fight" in the report of Covid prevention in China from BBC News, we found that in the limited usage of "fight", the "War" is depicted as between "individuals" and the "virus". 7 out of the 9 sentences that adopt the "War" metaphor using "fight" are painting a different scenario, in which the "fight" is not a "united fight" against the virus. Instead, there are kinds of "fight" described by the BBC News. All the types of separated "fights" are mentioned in BBC News, deliberately deconstructing the concept of a "united fight" between China as a whole against the virus. For example,

St. 11　That trains the **body to fight off the real virus** when it comes into contact with it.

St. 12　Made by CanSino, it has similar ingredients to its injected vaccine, using a harmless adenovirus as a carrier for the genetic code that teaches **the body how to fight Covid**.

The above two sentences depict the "fight" as solely between "individuals" and the virus.

Using "fight" literally rather than metaphorically is another approach to deconstruct the "War" metaphor commonly used to rationalize the prevention measures taken by China during the pandemic. BBC News reports on China's Covid prevention try to tear apart the "War" metaphor in describing China's fight against Covid-19 by using "fight" in different circumstances and by dividing the "united fight" into separate ones.

Interestingly, although BBC News is not willing to use "fight" in describing China's Covid prevention activities, it does use quite a few "War" metaphors to depict the situation. Only the emphasis is not on the "fighting" spirit, but on the usual strict control policies during wartime. As a result, we can find 9 sentences with the word "war", each of which is comparing China's Covid prevention as a "War". On the contrary, when we search for the word "War" in *China Daily*'s reports on China's Covid prevention, we find zero metaphorical expressions. Although *China Daily* used "Fight" frequently, which can activate the "War" metaphor framework in general, it seems that it is reluctant in claiming the "fight" against the virus an actual "war". It is more like a selected "War" metaphor, which only chooses part of the semantic molecules of "War", such as the merits of soldiers, including "persistence, determination, courage, and sacrifice".

Chapter 2 Corpus-Based Comparison of Disease Metaphors in English and Chinese

Meanwhile, other factors related to the period of war are backgrounded.

The "War" metaphor used by BBC News in explicating the Covid prevention in China highlights exactly the different semantic features of war. Instead of highlighting soldiers' merits, it focuses on the negative impact of "war" on common people's lives, including the "shortage of supplies, tightened restriction over movement, and the potential danger of losing". That is why the keyword "war" as a metaphorical expression for Covid prevention turns out to be more frequent in BBC News than in *China Daily*'s reports. Here are some example sentences including the "War" metaphors from BBC,

St. 13 Next to a paragraph describing increasing Chinese incomes and lifestyle changes since the country opened up in the 1970s, a text box mentions the "**war on Covid**".

St. 14 Beyond telling its own citizens that it has largely won the **war over its Covid-**19, China also wants to tell the world.

We can see from the above examples that BBC News is emphasizing on the possible negative impact of "War" on people's daily lives. It is doing so by collocating verbs with the "War" metaphor, creating a sense that "people" are suffering under the "war-like" scenario. In addition, they activate the "War" metaphor in a general level, leaving out the efforts and sacrifice China has made in buying more time for the other areas of the world to make plans in coping with the pandemic.

The analysis of "War" metaphor in the reports on Covid-19 in China from both BBC News and *China Daily* has shown us that the semantic frame and metaphorical themes used by the media can reflect their positions and perspectives. Even when the same metaphor is applied, the highlighted semantic molecules may differ, just as what we discussed above about the use of "War" metaphor. The same metaphorical theme can cause different reader reactions due to the context and the framework used in presenting the events. The "War" metaphor in *China Daily* is used to bring people together in the face of the common enemy—coronavirus, and to boost people's confidence and persistence in winning. On the other hand, when the same "War" metaphor is applied in BBC News, the highlighted features are the negative impact of war on people's lives in all aspects. While using "War" metaphor to boost people's morale and bring people together in a difficult time is the common practice in many countries, the attempt to separate its people from the government is hardly a common practice of all countries, but is limited to the Western developed countries who still hold on to the Cold War mindset and try to contain China's development even at a cost of themselves.

2.2.2 More Metaphorical Themes Involved in the Reports on Pandemic Prevention in *China Daily* and BBC News

After reading about 20 articles on Covid prevention in China from both *China Daily* and BBC News, about 10,000 words from each source, we have enriched the main metaphors mentioned in the above table. Apart from those mentioned in Table 2-6, more metaphorical themes used in the two sources are displayed in the following table.

Table 2-7 More conceptual metaphors used in the reports on Covid in China

Plants	Thrived, Sprung Up
Dark/Winter	Dark, winter, cold But during the dark winter of COVID, China hit the accelerator-adding as much wind power in two years as it had in the previous seven.
Wave/Stable/Up and down	Stabilize, ease, ensure, guarantee, peace Zhang Jiangbo, deputy director of the Department of Trade at the National Development and Reform Commission, spoke highly of the government's measures to ensure smooth logistics and its accelerated push for building a modern logistics system, saying it helps to **stabilize** the overall economy and promote healthy development amid the COVID-19 pandemic.
Fire	Resurgent, resurgence China's manufacturing activity contracted in April due to a **resurgence** in domestic COVID-19 infections coupled with uncertainties brought about by geopolitical tensions.
Engineering	One-size-fits-all Countries must consider their own realities and devise anti-virus policies that best suit their own situations; there is no **one-size-fits-all** approach.

In the above text, we have discussed the different highlights of "War" metaphors in BBC News and *China Daily*. Apart from "War" metaphor, another common metaphor used in describing the pandemic is the "Journey" metaphor, which perceives the pandemic as a "journey" we need to go through. "Journey" metaphor assumes a destined end to the pandemic, which can to some extent mitigate the suffering in the process. The representative key metaphor words for "journey" include "step", "direction", "move", as well as "emerge", which is usually used to depict the new situation during travelling. We used "step" as a keyword to search for the sentences that activate a "Journey" metaphor in describing Covid-19 or measures taken in curbing the virus. It turns out that both BBC News and *China Daily* use quite a few "step" words in their reports. However, albeit the similar activation of the "Journey" metaphors, the "journey" the two sources talk about are completely different. In the reports from *China Daily*, the "journey" we are on is definitely leading us to a better destination. And common phrases including "step" are "step up", "next step" and "solid, crucial or important" step. For example,

St. 15　China also proposed the convening of a committee as soon as possible to provide recommendations on the **next step** in long-term COVID-19 prevention and control, the delegate said.

St. 16　As China continues to take strict epidemic prevention and control measures, it has **taken solid steps** to smoothen transport and logistics services, and accelerate the building of a unified domestic market.

St. 17　As COVID-19 cases increase in many parts of the country, a number of educational institutions in China are **stepping up** their virus intervention efforts, The Paper reported.

It can be seen from the above examples that China is more future-oriented when it comes to Covid prevention and the recovery of economy in post-pandemic era. The phrases like "next step" and "step up" are used to boost readers' confidence in the future. Besides, the talks about the following "steps" also send out a message that the government has a plan, knows what to do, and is functioning according to the plan efficiently, which also adds lustre to the image of the government and sends out positive messages to the market. We can see that the "Journey" metaphor used in *China Daily* is more of a "promising journey" that leads us to a bright future. The "Promising journey" metaphor is also frequently activated when the topic goes on the economic development in the post-pandemic era, including the metaphor words "step", or other related words like "track", "direction", etc. For example,

St. 18 The dynamic prevention and control measures China has adopted, including lockdowns, mass testing and contact tracing, have kept the number of infections and deaths low while keeping the country's economic activities and people's livelihoods basically **on a normal track**, albeit with some inconvenience caused to local residents because of a sometimes rushed response by health officials in some COVID 19-hit places due to either mismanagement or a lack of capability.

St. 19 The integration of the Belt and Road Initiative with the new development plans of the Central Asian countries will be **an important step** in that direction.

St. 20 "In the **next step**, we will solidly implement these measures to ensure private investment volume and quality and give better play to private investment in promoting high-quality economic development," Gu said.

St. 21 It is also necessary to **step up efforts** in making proactive fiscal policy more effective and prudent monetary policy more targeted so as to create synergy for expanding demand.

No matter in the description of Covid prevention or in discussing the economic sectors, "Journey" metaphor is almost unanimously positive. The collocates for "steps" are either adjectives with a positive semantic prosody, such as "valid", "solid", "significant", "crucial", "important", or future-oriented prepositions like "up", "to", "towards". In order to better understand the context for "step" in *China Daily*'s report on Covid-19, we uploaded the collected reports into Sketch Engine as a mini Corpora, and searched for the collocates of "step" in the corpora. The top five collocates for "step" are shown in Table 2-8.

Table 2-8 Top 5 collocates for the "Journey" metaphor word "step" in *China Daily*

Word	Coocurrances	Candidates	T-Score	MI	LogDice
next	11	44	3.31	9.80	11.82
taken	6	40	2.44	9.06	11.00
up	17	278	4.10	7.77	10.70
efforts	8	149	2.81	7.58	10.32
practical	3	21	1.73	8.99	10.32

Different from the "promising journey" established in *China Daily*, the "journey" in BBC News is filled with uncertainty. By searching for the same keyword "step" for "Journey" metaphors, we have found the following example sentences:

St. 22   Again, for a country with an economy being smashed by Zero-Covid, **baby steps** are better than no steps.

St. 23   The moves announced today may not seem like much if you are not living in China but, inside the country, three years into a crisis, with no indication of when or how an **off ramp** may appear, any steps towards re-opening are **steps** which are not going backwards.

St. 24   Prof Huang believes there is a window between two highly politically sensitive events—the Olympics next month and the 20th Communist Party Congress at the end of the year—where China could take **steps** towards living with Covid.

We can see from the above example sentences from BBC News that there is hardly any positive or affirmative adjectives to modify the "steps". Besides, in St. 23 and 24, although no negative modifiers are used to depict the "steps", the steps are placed in an uncertain environment featured by words like "crisis", "no indication" and modal verbs like "could". Rather than a "promising" journey with ensured bright destination, the "journey" painted by BBC News is a "frustrating" journey with anxiety and uncertainty. We also searched for the frequent collocates for the word "step" in the reports of China's Covid situation from BBC News, and the top 5 collocates are shown in the following table.

Table 2-9   Top 5 collocates for the "Journey" metaphor word "step" in BBC News

Word	Concurrences	Candidates	T-Score	MI	LogDice
towards	6	18	2.45	9.99	11.46
down	13	154	3.59	8.01	11.01
surveillance	4	22	2.00	9.12	10.79
up	14	219	3.72	7.61	10.73
major	3	82	1.72	6.80	9.52
to	14	3741	3.41	3.51	6.92

By contrasting Table 2-8 and Table 2-9, we can observe that in the "Journey" metaphor from BBC News, "step down" ranks higher than "step up" according to

MI and LogDice, while among the top 5 collocates for "step" in *China Daily*'s reports, "Next" is preferred over "up". The contrast supports our argument above that the "journey" depicted by *China Daily* is more "promising" and future-oriented, while the "journey" in the eyes of BBC News is more pessimistic and gloomy. Besides, the main adjective used to describe "step" in *China Daily* is practical, while the main modifier for "step" in BBC News is "surveillance". The contrast in the semantic prosody of these two words also demonstrates the different emphasis in "Journey" metaphors between the two sources.

Another key metaphor word for the conceptual "Journey" metaphor is "move". After searching for the word "move" in the two corpora, we are able to locate 86 hits of "move" in BBC News, and 43 hits of "move" in *China Daily*. Apparently, "move" is a preferred word in metaphorically describing government policies in BBC News, especially when the country concerned is China. Semantically, the word "move" is a neutral word, indicating the change of location in its basic meaning, while it is usually used to refer to the plan for future of an individual or of a country. In fact, the overall "Journey" metaphor is built on the conceptual metaphor that LIFE IS A JOURNEY. And the metaphor is applied to describe the development of a country when we personify a country's development as a person's growth. Therefore, the "move" of a country also activates the "Journey" metaphor in general. However, in BBC's report on China's dealing with Covid-19, the direction for China's "move" is either "away" or "from" something and path, or being stagnant or stuck when other countries have moved on.

In the "Journey" metaphor activated by the word "move" in BBC News, China is either "not moving" when others are, or is "moving away from", from BBC News. The reports highlight the struggling and difficulty for China to "move". It is actually quite interesting to look at the use of "Journey" metaphor when BBC News is reporting China. It almost feels that Western media like BBC News are afraid of talking about China's future in an objective tone. Thus they refuse to discuss this topic by blocking the "journey" with "not moving" or by pouring suspicion, uncertainty and anxiety to the "journey" ahead of China to damp down the energetic and lively vibe, and turn the "journey" into a bleak and grim one. On the contrary, in the 43 hits of "move" in *China Daily*, after the verbal or nominal "move", there is always a "destination" or "direction" that follows. Each "move" is aimed at a new goal, and each "move" represents a "move" forward, a "move" to bring the country to a better place in the long "journey".

St. 25　Perhaps China should focus more on other areas and potential threats to transform and upgrade traditional industries, and foster and expand strategic emerging industries, while **moving industries to the medium-high end**, he said.

St. 26　He stressed the need for efforts to improve purchasing policies for recovery is strengthening people's confidence in development, the premier said, stressing the importance of **moving the manufacturing industry toward high-end, green and smart development**.

St. 27　Another **move to strengthen industry chains** is developing characteristic towns with advantageous local specialty industries.

St. 28　"China is at a critical stage of **moving from being a manufacturing powerhouse to a smart-manufacturing center**, which will generate more opportunities," Yang said at the company's global suppliers conference in Tianjin.

To the opposite of the "move" illustrated by BBC News, the "move" in *China Daily* is always "forward" and purpose-oriented. The journey activated by the word "move" is guaranteed and ensured, and the aim of the "move" is made loud and clear. In the scenario described in *China Daily*, each "move" is made with a clear aim in mind. Similar to the "journey" activated by "step", each "move" is made with firm belief and confidence. While "step" lays more on the efficiency side, "move" is used to indicate that the "direction" is right. The same characteristics can also be identified in the usage of the word "direction", which is also a "trigger" word for the "Journey" metaphors. Similar to the use of "step" and "move", when "direction" is applied in *China Daily*'s reports on China, the main modifiers for "direction" are "positive", "important", and "of high efficiency", which are ensuring an "upward" direction for a "promising journey". For example,

St. 29　... expected to form a virtuous circle step by step, and guide market expectation, confidence and capital in the **positive direction**, Yao said.

Cognitive and Contrastive Analysis of Disease Metaphors in English and Chinese

St. 30 ... believes cultural cooperation between both sides will continue, and joint restoration work will become an **important direction for their future cooperation**.

St. 31 The plan required upgrading the traditional industries like coal mining, steelmaking and machinery toward the **directions of higher efficiency** and cleaner and safer operations.

However, the same word "direction" sounds more negative and uncertain when it is used in the reports on China from BBC News. As shown in the following sentence:

St. 32 ... like the idea of reducing foreign influence in China, and the pandemic has provided an excellent excuse to move **in this direction**.

Besides, the searching results of the metaphor word "path" help us understand another enhanced semantic molecules of "Journey" metaphor, that is, the common "path" for mankind as a community with shared future. It is not about asking another country to switch their own "path" to another one. Instead, it is asking the world to take a perspective that transcends the national angle. Despite the differences in culture and ethnic identities, we are all human beings living on the same planet, thus there are common interests between all the countries, like the development of science and technology to better treat diseases, and the protection of the environment, and the control of climate change.

St. 33 Craig Allen, president of the US-China Business Council, said via video link that joint efforts should be made to ensure that both countries **consent to a path** on which competitive concerns do not outplay beneficial cooperation.

St. 34 The China-proposed **Belt and Road Initiative is a prime example of such win-win intent** and project.

St. 35 "G7 members to catch up with the trend of the times, focus on addressing the various issues they have at home, stop ganging up to form exclusive blocs, stop containing and bludgeoning other countries, stop creating and stoking bloc confrontation and get back to the **right path of dialogue and cooperation**," said the spokesperson.

Chapter 2　Corpus-Based Comparison of Disease Metaphors in English and Chinese

It can be seen from the above examples that the "journey" described in *China Daily* is not confined to one country alone, but rather a negotiated road for multiple countries based on consent. It is not asking all the other countries to adopt the "path" of China, but is saying that different countries can always find a common "path" to realize win-win results through communication and cooperation. China has always been open and holds an inclusive mindset towards different cultures and political systems. However, Western media like BBC News is stuck with the Cold War mindset. In their reports, the activated "Journey" metaphor is doomed to end nowhere simply because it is not the same with their "path" of modernization and development. And they are used to take the moral high ground and judge China's way within their culture, and criticize China's actions whenever it contradicts their definition of the so-called "universal value".

Besides, while the "Journey" metaphor activated in BBC's reports only on China, and adopted a gloomy and bleak shade, the "journey" talked about in *China Daily* is not limited to China alone, but related to the future development of the world and mankind as a whole. As an emerging large economy in the world, China assumes more international responsibilities and is not only concerned with its prospect. To the opposite, BBC's report on China focuses all its attention on China alone, ignoring China's essential role in driving the world economy and helping the underdeveloped areas to develop and prosper.

Another theme of higher metaphoricity within the reports on China from *China Daily* is "Location and direction", which is the combination of "Spatial-temporal" conceptual metaphor and the "Journey" metaphor, laying more stress on the spatial conceptualization of the current situation or status of China and its future development. Typical words used to designate the current situation of China are "position", "stood", "center", "position", "destination", and "located". Besides, the representative metaphor words to symbolize the "journey" China is walking on is "direction" and "destination". We have provided some example sentences for "direction". As to "destination", it is frequently used to refer to the "goal" in economic development, the advancement of investment promotion, and the furthering of community with shared future for mankind.

To sum up, although the "Journey" metaphor is adopted in both *China Daily* and BBC News, the highlighted features are quite different. In the description of

China Daily, the "journey" China is on is a promising journey with an ensured brighter destination, the current hardship and inconvenience will definitely pay off in the long run. However, the "journey" depicted in BBC News is filled with "uncertainty" and "unknown", it is almost a "journey" that will undoubtedly lead to a dead end. Thus China is expected to "divert" from the current path sooner or later, and the current hardship will be more likely to continue unless there is a change of "direction". The assurance of the "journey" results in more positive energy in *China Daily*'s reports, while the questioning and challenging of the "journey" leads to more negative interpretation of what is going on in China during and after the pandemic.

So far we have introduced two major metaphors used in both *China Daily* and BBC News: "War" metaphor and "Journey" metaphor. And through the comparison and examples from each source, we understand that the two sources have their own choices of highlighted features albeit both are employing the same general conceptual metaphor framework. The fact that both sources are using the same metaphor to highlight completely different features is a demonstration that metaphor is a matter of selection, and it can send out various messages based on what is your focus of attention and what is the information that is backgrounded. Besides the frequent use of "War" metaphor and "Journey" metaphor, another three metaphors are also commonly used in the reports on China during the pandemic from *China Daily*, they are the "Vehicle and inland transport" metaphor and the "Sailing and swimming" metaphor, both of them are laying emphasis on the energetic and dynamic developing trend in China. Besides, another metaphor is the "Person" metaphor, which turns out to be a relative frequent metaphor in both *China Daily* and BBC News, the same as "War" metaphor and "Journey" metaphor, the two sources are again using the same "Person" metaphor in different ways. Now let us look at these interesting metaphors in the following text, together with some example sentences to illustrate how the metaphors are activated.

Through the comparison of the two articles from both *China Daily* and BBC News, we have learned that BBC News tends to use more "Person" metaphors to describe China. On the contrary, *China Daily* prefers to see China as a united power against the enemy, the "War" metaphor is frequently activated. Apart from depicting China as a strong and united "troop" or "soldier", the Wmatix semantic

Chapter 2 Corpus-Based Comparison of Disease Metaphors in English and Chinese

tagging of the collected 320 articles from *China Daily* has revealed more metaphorical themes used to describe China. For example, when the topic is about China's economic recovery or development, "Tough/Strong" is a repeated theme.

St. 36   Industry insiders said China, the world's second-largest fuel consumer, has led the world in oil demand recovery, with its economy displaying **strong resilience**.

St. 37   China's economy expanded 8.1 percent year-on-year with major indicators reaching the expected targets, showcasing its **strong resilience** and vitality despite the impact of the COVID-19 pandemic, officials and experts said on Monday.

The above examples examplify the "strong player" image of China in the economic field, which echoes the tough "soldier" image mentioned in the above text within the "War" metaphor in discussing the pandemic. Besides, another intriguing metaphorical theme from the semantic tagging analysis is "Vehicle and transport on land". A further look into the example sentences of this theme reveals the common metaphor of China's economy as the "transport on land", especially "the engine of the vehicle". For example,

St. 38   We are evolving quickly to become a global green energy, green metals and green hydrogen business to **drive** the de-carbonization of the aviation, mining, steel and fertilizer industry.

St. 39   But during the dark winter of COVID, China hit the **accelerator** adding as much wind power in two years as it had in the previous seven.

St. 40   On the other hand, a long-term optimistic outlook can stem from a combination of new and old economic **drivers** as China focuses on stabilizing growth.

From the above examples, we can learn that the economic and technological development is frequently compared to "vehicles and transport on land". The highlighted common feature between the two domains is "the fast speed", and the established scenario includes the vechile that is driving fast on the road, symbolizing the fast-developing economy of technology in China. The "Vehicle and transport on land" theme is closely related to the above-mentioned "Journey/Path" theme, since the condition of the "road" ensures the fast speed of the "vehicle", and direction the "path" leads to determine if the "vehicle" can reach the expected destination. More example sentences include the "Journey/Path" metaphor that is closely associated with the "Vehicle" metaphor are shown as follows,

St. 41　The GBF serves as a comprehensive **road map** for global action on biodiversity conservation.

St. 42　Liu Qingfeng, chairman of Chinese artificial intelligence pioneer iFlytek Co, said the nation is **on the right track** to joining the top ranks in the world in terms of technological innovation.

So far, we have listed the two interesting thematic metaphors revealed through the semantic tagging of Wmtrix towards the articles collected from *China Daily*. Apart from a "strong player" and the "vehicle or transport on land", another two interesting metaphors are the "Sailing and swimming" metaphor and the "Darkness" metaphor. The "Sailing and swiming" theme is reflected by the repetition of words like "flow", "dive", "launch", "anchor" and "wake (the trace left by the ship)". The metaphor is built on the similarities between the connection of different "products", "resources", "knowledge" and "ideas" with the continuousness of water. Similar to the flowing water, the connection between the "products", "resources", "knowledge" and "ideas" is expected to be so smooth that the movement or the transportation of them resembles the non-stopping flowing water. The highlighted common features in the process is the continuousness and smoothiness of the transportation of resources or the communication of ideas. For example,

St. 43　Further modernized system seen as key to propelling development amid COVID China's intensified efforts to build a modern logistics system will help facilitate the **smooth flow of products and resources**, boost economic circulation and stabilize growth amid downward pressure, officials and experts said.

St. 44　She has reasons for that declaration she **dived** into the capital market upon graduating from the university by buying some money market products.

St. 45　We will make more efforts to optimize the open innovation ecosystem and promote the **smooth flow** of knowledge, technology and talent, in order to provide a broader stage for international scientific and technological organizations, scientists, entrepreneurs and investors to come to China for innovation and business expansion, Wang said.

St. 46　In 2017, China **launched** the Digital Silk Road, adding a new dimension to the Belt and Road Initiative.

St. 47　The one-China principle is the **solid anchor** for peace and stability in the Taiwan Strait.

St. 48　Need to boost domestic high-technology sector Sovereign wealth funds in the Gulf region are also increasing their holdings in China, indicating increasing **capital flow** into China.

St. 49　Muhammad Hasanein Khaddam, Syrian ambassador to China, said China "stood out as an exemplary case of humanity **in the wake of** the COVID-19 pandemic".

St. 50　The legendary route activated more than 2,000 years ago bore witness to interactions between China and Central Asia through tradings of merchandise and **flows of ideas**.

In St. 43, 45, 48 and 50, we can observe that "products and resources", "knowledge, technology and talent", "capital" and "ideas" are all modified by the metaphorical word "flow", as if all of these things are capable of "flowing" from one place to another like a "river", emphasizing the convenience in transportation and the efficiency in communication. St. 46, 47 and 50 are also related to sailing, either the initiation of the "Silk Road" or the "anchoring" of peace and stability, both are painting the picture of a "sailing boat". The boat has kept moving forward despite the fluctuating waves caused by Covid-19, and it can sail steadily on the surface of the ocean. Different from the "Vehicle and transport on land" metaphor, which prioritizes the speed of development, the "Swimming and sailing" metaphor attaches importance to the close connections between things and ideas. When "Vehicle and transport on land" mainly emphasizes the development in economic and technological fields, the "Swimming and sailing" metaphor highlights international cooperation in various domains.

In addition, another interesting metaphor used mainly in describing the pandemic period and the US policies that aim to contain China's development is

Cognitive and Contrastive Analysis of Disease Metaphors in English and Chinese

"Darkness". As we know, China persists in fighting the virus through lockdown and quarantine when most of the Western countries have given up. Due to the fact that Chinese government has chosen a different way in the prevention of Covid-19, there have been many voices from the West. From the reports of Covid in *China Daily*, we can notice that "Darkness" is used to describe the bleak period when people are facing the threat of coronavirus. Besides, "Dark" is also used to modify the despicable behavior of the United Sates in containing other countries' development and in its coercive diplomacy. Example sentences to illustrate the "Darkness" metaphor can be seen as follows,

St. 51　But during the **dark winter of COVID**, China hit the accelerator—adding as much wind power in two years as it had in the previous seven.

St. 52　Today, we see this **dark history** being repeated. Facing economic and social problems in the US, then President Barack Obama adopted the Pivot to Asia policy in 2011, targeting China's rise with a containment policy of military expansion and economic isolation.

Another distinctive semantic theme that is prominent among the themes of *China Daily*'s reports on China during the pandemic is "Architecture, houses and buildings". This theme enjoys a higher relative frequency of 0.31%, while the relative frequency value in BBC written is 0.27%, meaning that this theme is overused in O1 (the dataset collected from *China Daily*). However, the same theme is even not found in the reports on China from BBC News. By going over the concordance of this theme, we identified the main representative words, such as "build", "construct", "bridge", "apartment", "properties", "scaffold", "architecture". Among these words, different forms of the word "build" are used more frequently. Therefore, to better understand the collocates of the representative metaphor word "build" of the "Architecture, houses and buildings" theme, we searched for the keyword "build" in the self-created corpus of *China Daily*'s reports on China during the pandemic on Sketch Engine. The top 10 collocates of the word "build" are displayed in the following table.

Chapter 2 Corpus-Based Comparison of Disease Metaphors in English and Chinese

Table 2-10 Top 10 collocates of "build" in the corpus of *China Daily*'s reports on China

No.	Words	Cooccurrances	Candidates	T-Score	MI	LogDice
1	community	20	89	4.46	8.09	11.34
2	modern	13	37	3.60	8.74	11.05
3	logistics	10	64	3.15	7.57	10.49
4	portfolios	6	6	2.45	10.25	10.18
5	China-Central	9	99	2.97	6.79	10.13
6	system	10	148	3.12	6.36	10.04
7	strength	5	14	2.23	8.76	9.85
8	together	6	50	2.43	7.19	9.84
9	platform	6	65	2.43	6.81	9.75
10	China-Africa	4	13	1.99	8.55	9.53

It can be seen from Table 2-10 that the most frequent collocate for "build" is "community", which refers to "the community with a shared future for mankind". Apart from "community", words like "China-Central" and "China-Africa" are also attaching importance to the establishment of harmonious international relations with Central Asia countries and African countries, who are all member states of the developing countries. The priority of "cooperation" between these countries are examples to prove that China indeed aims to build the shared community for mankind instead of the old mindset guided by zero-sum game. The top 10 collocates also provide us with a more specific understanding of the "building" China intends to "construct". "The community with shared future for mankind" is examplified with the "building" of global community of health for all, the modern logistics and industrial system to facilitate the exchange of products, and the financing portforlios to help boost the economic prosperity through South-and-South cooperation. The "construction" of the "community" also requires China to "build up" its strength in industry, agricultural modernization, and in cultural confidence. Moreover, "the community with shared future for mankind" can not be "built" by China alone. It can only be built together by friendly countries who share the same value. Representative metaphors of the "Architecture, houses and buildings" theme can be found in the following example sentences:

St. 53 ... pledges to offer international aid to boost developing countries' pandemic response, calling for the world to build **a global community of health** for all, during his speech by video link in Beijing on Friday to the Global Health Summit.

St. 54 He pointed out that the efforts between both sides in building **a community of common development and security** have seen "encouraging progress" over the past four years.

St. 55 Further modernized system seen as key to propelling development amid COVID China's intensified efforts to **build a modern logistics system** will help facilitate the smooth flow of products and resources, boost economic circulation.

The frequent usage of "Architecture, houses and building" thematic metaphor in describing China's policies during the pandemic serves as a reflection of the positive attitude of China in the face of hardship. Even during the pandemic, when the country is concentrating on overcoming the difficulties posed by the virus, Chinese government still holds on to strategic and constructive thinking: How can the world better cope with the next pandemic? What can make the mankind safer and stronger? What is the solution to the economic downturn caused by the pandemic? The upbeat and positive perspective of the Chinese government allows it to focus more on the future opportunities to make the world a better place through cooperation, instead of "pointing fingers" and accusing others for the outbreak of the pandemic or for not handling the disease in the way expected by certain countries. Each country has its own domestic situation, and it should be up to the government and the people of the independent country to decide what is the best measure in coping with the pandemic.

On the contrary, the searching results of "build" in the corpus of BBC's reports show a completely different scenario. There are actually very few metaphors involved, and "build" is used mainly in its literal sense, like "build" the "anti-epidemic barrier", "more hospital ICU", and the "production plant" or "a brand new" city. The lack of "Architecture, houses and buildings" theme in the reports on China from BBC News implicates its reluctance in talking about China's situation in a constructive way.

Chapter 2   Corpus-Based Comparison of Disease Metaphors in English and Chinese

Apart from "Architecture, houses and buildings", another distinctive theme from *China Daily*'s reports on China is "Children's games and toys", represented by metaphor words like "player and jigsaw". The metaphorical usage of "players" illustrates a scenario that visualizes the world as a big stage or playground, in which different countries play their roles on the stage. For example,

St. 56   As nations grapple with the devastating consequences of climate change, the Association of Southeast Asian Nations and China have emerged as **key players** in fostering a green transformation.

St. 57   The country's space agency, the China National Space Administration (CNSA), has made significant strides in recent years, signaling its intent to become a **formidable player** in the cosmic quest.

St. 58   More and more **global players** in different sectors eye the huge advantages of the Zhongguancun area, and choose to create in China for the world.

St. 59   As the second-largest economy in the world, China has been playing a constructive role in the global economy by being a **multilateral player**.

St. 60   One initiative in the province is to foster 10 competitive industry chains through backing dozens of **leading players** in these sectors.

In all of the above examples, we can learn that *China Daily* recognizes the fact that nowadays the world is seeing the emergence of multiple players. The multi-polarization of the world in both economy and politics is an unstoppable trend. Besides, there is no denying that China is now a key player in the international stage, as the second largest economy in the world. Viewing the world as a playground with all the countries live and play harmoniously in the playground. Each "player" can benefit from the cooperation and communication between different countries.

The argument that the Western countries refuse to recognize a stronger China as a key player in the international stage is supported by the lack of "Game" metaphor in BBC's reports on China. It seems that in the eyes of the Western media, China does not count as a "player" in their circle. Exactly because they refuse to put aside their prejudice, bias and stereotype of China, they began to fear the development and the rise of China. Thus instead of "Game" metaphors, we have semantic themes like "Constraint", "Hindering" and "Danger" ranked relatively higher among all the semantic themes. Taking the "Danger" as an example, we can find sentences that include words like "risk", as in "China's big risk now is removing Covid restrictions without having a broadly vaccinated population", and "pitfalls", as in "Pitfalls lie ahead as China exits zero-Covid", as well as words like "dangerous", "gambling", "unsafe", "exposure" and "precarious". However, the theme "Danger" is not found in the reports on China from *China Daily*.

On the contrary, we have found the opposite theme "Safe" and "Safety/Danger" which enjoys a high ranking among all the semantic themes. It is quite interesting when the two media view the situation in China from such contradictory viewpoints. While BBC News sees China with a rather pessimistic perspective, highlighting the "risks" and "dangers" that may pose threat to the country during and after the pandemic, *China Daily* has more faith in China's proper handling of the situation and providing a safe environment for its people. For example, under the "Safe" and "Safety/Danger" theme, we have example sentences that include words like "safe", as in "The plan shows a modern distribution system that is safe, reliable and highly efficient with a global reach", and "safety", as in "China will comprehensively strengthen production safety of the marine fishery sector", as well as "safeguard", as in "continue to improve mechanisms for maintaining national security to better safeguard prosperity and development".

Moreover, another contradictory theme to "Safety" is "Fear/Shock", represented by words like "fear", "panic", "shock", "alarm", "frightened", "menace", "fearsome", "horrors" and "terrifying". Among them the word "fear" enjoys 87 hits in the collected articles from BBC News. To better understand how "fear" is presented, and what kind of metaphors are involved in describing "fear", we also searched for the word "fear" in the self-established corpus made of articles from BBC in Sketch Engine. The collocation analysis is shown in the following table.

Chapter 2 Corpus-Based Comparison of Disease Metaphors in English and Chinese

Table 2-11 Top 10 collocates of "fear" in the corpus of BBC's reports on China

No.	Words	Cooccurrances	Candidates	T-Score	MI	LogDice
1	fury	12	15	3.46	10.51	11.91
2	spark	10	13	3.16	10.45	11.68
3	self-infect	9	9	3.00	10.83	11.58
4	amid	10	56	3.15	8.35	11.16
5	over	15	260	3.84	6.72	10.47
6	freedom	4	15	2.00	8.93	10.33
7	from	4	21	1.99	8.44	10.25
8	drove	3	5	1.73	10.09	10.06
9	deaths	10	221	3.12	6.37	10.06
10	Covid	22	1,201	4.55	5.06	9.13

It can be seen from Table 2-11 that the "fury and fear" is a frequent phrase used in BBC's reports on China during the pandemic, establishing the solemn and desolate scenario. Among the two words, "spark" is usually used in front of the word "fear". The other collocates of the word "fear" can be classified into two groups. One group focuses on the question "who is in fear" and the other question deals with the question "fear what". By giving the "who" and "what", the "fear" can become more concrete and real, contributing to the fostering of a bleak atmosphere.

Together with "Fear/Shock", another distinctive negative themes that are opposite to the frequent themes like "Helping" and "Safety" are "Worry" and "Violent/Angry". Both "Worry" and "Violent/Angry" are exclusive themes to BBC New's reports on China. Within these two themes, "Worry" is featured by words like "concerns", "worried", "desperation", "worry", "disturbing", "anxious", "anxiety", "ordeal", "distress". Meanwhile, "Violence/Angry" is demonstrated with words like "anger", "hit", "fury", "angry", "threaten", "unrest", "clashes", "force", "outrage", "attack", "aggressive", "violence", "abuse", "outburst", "raged", "ferocious". Taking "concern" and "anger" as examples, we searched for their collocates in the corpus on Sketch Engine. It is found that the top collocate for "concern" is "raised", while the top collocate for "anger" is "desperation". For example, according to the searching results, there are "raised concerns" about "cause of death", "misinformation", and over "the vaccination rate", "the disruption of the supply chain", "China's ability in maintaining the zero-covid policy". All of these examples prove the constant biased attitude of BBC when it comes to "what happened in China". Just like the "underworld filter" preferred by the BBC News in presenting different places in China, they cling to this biased and suspicious attitude in almost all of their reports on China. BBC News was really good at and was getting used to treating themselves as the "representative loudspeaker" for Chinese people based on the information they dug out from the Internet, mainly the social media. Without confirming the source of the news, they would rush to the negative interpretation or conclusion based on their inherent stereotype of China.

2.3 Further Analysis of Contradictory Themes from Two Sources

So far, we have discussed several contradictory themes in the reports on China from *China Daily* and BBC News. In fact, there are more contrary pairs between the two sources. We summarized those opposite theme pairs in Table 2-12.

Table 2-12 Contrary semantic themes from *China Daily* and BBC News

Themes from *China Daily*	Representative Words	Contrary Themes from BBC News	Representative Words
Helping	support, help, boost, assist, facilitate, promote ...	Constraint	restriction, lock, detain, confine, contain, limit ...
Safety/ Danger	safe, safety, safeguard ...	Danger/ Fear & shock/ Worry/Violent & anger	risk, danger, threat, fear, concern, anger, raged, unrest, anxious, clash ...
Evaluation: Good/Bad	good, improve, promote, reliable, progress, enhance ...	Evaluation: Bad	worst, disaster, case scenario ...
Interested/ Excited/ Energetic	energy, spur, vigorous, dynamic, vitality, interest, incentive, proactive ...	Sad/Discontent	frustration, fed-up, disappoint, dissatisfaction, mourned ...

(continuous)

Themes from *China Daily*	Representative Words	Contrary Themes from BBC News	Representative Words
Sensory: Taste	taste	Sensory: Sight	see, watch, witness, observe, glimpse, spot, scan, glance, visibility ...
Success	thrived, winning, solving, defeat, effectiveness, successful, overcome, on track, achievement, beat, breakthrough, live up to, fruitful, flourished, producing ...	Failure	lost, failure, failed, losing, vain, down-the-drain, on-its-knee, bungling, went-wrong, blew it ...
Giving/ Finding/ Showing	provide, offer, supply, present, distribute, show, indicate, reflect, point out, display, exhibit ...	Putting/ Pulling/Pushing	place, put, bring, send, life, remove, suspend, stuck, deliver, take away, push, turn, throw, deploy, damp, steer ...

Table 2-12 presents the contrary semantic themes from *China Daily* and BBC News. We have already discussed the first three pairs in the previous text. Now let us look at the remaining opposite themes adopted in these two media agencies. There are two pairs related to human, both the emotion of human beings and the senses of humans. A clear contrast can be found in the expressed emotions in the reports from two sources. The persona depicted in *China Daily* is an upbeat individual filled with energy and enthusiasm, while the one illustrated in BBC News is a pessimistic and frustrated figure. By looking into the contexts of these words, we can discover that those modifiers are mainly used to describe China as a country, which can be seen as a type of ontological metaphors since we are personifying inanimate entities.

Despite the similar metaphorical mechanism adopted in describing the situation in China, the emotion that is transferred to the country differs. For example, in the reports from *China Daily*, we can find example sentences like "Thursday saw investors launching a spirited attempt to recover lost ground", and verbs like "spur" with objects like "the development of logistics", "growth opportunities", "market confidence" and "market vitality", as well as "global economic growth". Besides, the modifier "vigorous" is also used to enhance the impression that China is an energetic "person" with strong motive to prosper. For example, we can find sentences like "government's vigorous measures" and "the supply will remain vigorous".

Apart from the clear contrast between "Safety" and "Danger", we can also observe the contrast in "Evaluation". The reports on China from *China Daily* are featured by "good evaluation", demonstrated by words like "good", "great", "improve", "reliable", "upgrading", "progress", "high-quality", "favorable", "enhance". To the opposite, reports on China from BBC News have four "Evaluation" themes, which are "bad", "true", "false" subsequently, and none of the three "Evaluation" themes is positive. Within the "Evaluation: bad" theme, we can locate words like "worst", "disaster", "worst-case scenario", and the keywords in "Evaluation: false" theme are "distorting", "lie", "disinformation", "untrue", and "concoction". It is worth noticing that the use of the word "concoction" is classified within the "Evaluation: false" theme. Looking into the context for the word "concoction", we learn that it actually refers to the Traditional Chinese Medicine (TCM). The full sentence is "TCM is one of the world's oldest forms of medical practice and includes a range of treatments from herbal concoctions to acupuncture to Tai Chi." Even the topic is concerned with TCM, which is a traditional medical practice in China that enjoys a long history, the purposeful choice of the word "concoction" is pragmatically negative and implies that the "herbal mixture" is not reliable. This single example, together with the lack of "good evaluation" terms in BBC News can reflect the general negative attitude and the unfair evaluation of China in BBC's reports.

As to the "Evaluation" theme from *China Daily*, similar to the term label "Safety/Danger", the "Evaluation" theme is also labeled as "Evaluation: good/bad" for the examples given by *China Daily*, justifying that *China Daily* is adopting more neutral and objective evaluative words in discussing the situation in China, rather than focusing only on good sides or bad sides. For example, within the "Evaluation: good/bad" theme, we have neutral words like "standard", "quality", "ranking", "rating", and "ups and downs". As in the sentence

Chapter 2 Corpus-Based Comparison of Disease Metaphors in English and Chinese

"Industry experts agreed the way ahead may see ups and downs as the market pursues an overall recovery." Both "good" and "bad" evaluation can be found in the labeled semantic themes from *China Daily*.

Another interesting contrary metaphor is also a type of ontological metaphor. Instead of bequeathing the non-human entities, in this case, what's been transferred is the basic senses of the mankind. Among the five basic senses, we find the "taste" sense is used more in the reports on China from *China Daily*, while "sight" is a much popular sense adopted in BBC News. In order to better understand these two sensory metaphors, let us take a look at some example sentences of the "sight" sense first:

St. 61   However, there is no end in **sight** to China's existing measures.

St. 62   "The pandemic has certainly left something behind, even if it is not **visible** on the surface," one resident, Han Meimei, told the BBC.

Apart from "see" and "witness", words like "sight" and "visible" are appealing to the "sight". The use of words like "no ending sight" and "not visible" are also meant to bring more uncertainty and influence people with anxiety on the created uncertainties. The whole narrative assumes a gloomy and depressed tone as if one is placed in a controlled box without any future prospect. It seems to be an objective observation, but it is in fact a biased assumption pretending to be neutral.

The reason why "notice" is not favored in the reports on China from BBC News partly goes to the fact that "notice" and "look at" connote more agency compared with "see" and "witness". Indeed, the searching results for the verb "notice" in BBC's reports on China show us that "notice" is usually reserved for BBC observers or journalists, for example, "Driving along the road we noticed fresh mounds of earth with red flags placed on the top." Besides, another occasion that notice is used as a verb is in negative form, as in "Very little notice is often given before a lockdown, often triggering anger and anxiety." The choice of verbs in the "sensory" metaphor group almost deprives Chinese people of their ability in thinking on themselves and making their own "notice". It reflects the inherent arrogance of the West in assuming the high-end of both morality and intelligence. On the other hand, the Western media like BBC News is paying their sympathy to

Cognitive and Contrastive Analysis of Disease Metaphors in English and Chinese

the "pathetic" Chinese people who have no idea about what is going to happen to them. This twisted mindset may feed to the ego of some people of the Western world, who still live in the bubbles of dream and have no idea about the reality in modern China. Although not favored by the BBC News, "notice" and "noticeable" is frequently used in the "Seen" semantic theme of *China Daily*. For example,

St. 63 During the COVID-19 pandemic, Zeiss said it **noticed** people spending much longer hours on their electronic devices such as mobile phones.

St. 64 **Having noticed** that China's consumer-focused Internet is gradually transforming into a more business-oriented Internet, Wang said the modern logistics system will become key in supporting the country's economic transition and industrial restructuring.

Different from the sole emphasis on "sight", represented by words like "see" and "witness", *China Daily*'s reports on China do not have many metaphors devoted to only one sense. The only sensory metaphor located is related to "taste", which is not used in describing anything related to the pandemic. The taste metaphor is found in sentences like "She thinks the motto of the festival youthful passion, academic taste and cultural awareness distinguishes it clearly from others.", and another sentence that describes "tea", as in "Tea helps us sip the taste of life, enjoy the spiritual tranquility, evoke enlightenment, and bring our heart and soul back to mother nature".

There is also clear contrast between the theme "Success" and "Failure". In the first place, we need to make clear that in the reports on China from both *China Daily* and BBC News, we can locate both the theme of "Success and failure". *China Daily*'s reports do not have an independent semantic theme that is labeled "Failure", while there is indeed an independent "Failure" theme in BBC's reports on China. Going over the representative words and phrases within the themes of "Success" and "Success and failure", we have revealed several different metaphors in *China Daily*'s reports. One main conceptual metaphor is the "Plant" metaphor, of which China is seen as a growing plant or tree, especially when the topic goes about China's economy. There are metaphor words like "thrived", "fruitful", and "flourishing". Apart from the "Plant" metaphor, we can also find

Chapter 2　Corpus-Based Comparison of Disease Metaphors in English and Chinese

the "Journey" metaphor and the "Manufacturing or engineering" metaphor from words like "on track" and "breakthrough", as well as "producing". The phrase "live up to" is a combination of ontological spatial metaphor and the LIFE IS A JOURNEY metaphor, of which "Up" stands for "Good", and "living a meaningful life" resembles "walking on an upward journey". The fact that a higher density of metaphors are employed in describing "Success" in the reports of *China Daily* reflects that China and Chinese people do attach lots of importance to "being successful", and are proud of their achievements and the progress made in the process of China's development in all aspects. On the contrary, the words used under the theme "Failure" in BBC's report contain more "Animal" metaphors. For example, the word "bungle" is closely associated with the image of a "bear". Besides, the phrase "on-its-knee" is also a typical gesture when a person fails the battle.

The fact that China uses more "Plant" metaphors in describing success is in line with the peaceful nature of Chinese culture. The deep-rooted Chinese value firmly believes that one's success is rooted in one's own thriving and prospering, rather than winning over someone else or beating someone up. In other words, Chinese path of development does not lead to hegemony, for the best environment for a "tree" to grow is a "forest" where all the other trees are also thriving and blooming. The most used conceptual metaphor for "success" is a "thriving tree", which poses no threat to the surroundings. On the contrary, each "growing tree" can contribute to the construction of a balanced ecology. The better the ecological environment is, the better the trees grow. That is also why at many high-end international conferences, the Chinese voice is always affirming the possibility of win-win, and the establishment of a harmonious community with shared future for mankind.

Besides, since the "Plant" metaphor is the dominant metaphor when Chinese people think of both the success of an individual and the prosperity of a nation, the correspondent mindset and value for most Chinese people is that one needs to take root in the deep ground and absorb the nutrition as much as possible to grow taller so as to get enough sunshine. The key is to rely on one's own efforts rather than taking up others' ground. And when there are disputes or conflicts, China's traditional culture makes people believe that one should first reflect on one's own actions or behaviors instead of pointing fingers at others. Therefore, the popularity of "Plant" metaphors in *China Daily*'s reports under the theme "Success" reflects the peaceful nature of Chinese culture.

However, different from the popularity of the "Plant" metaphor in the description of success, the main metaphor used under the "Success" theme in BBC's reports on China is the "Fight" and "Race" metaphor. The representative metaphor words for the "Fight" metaphor are "beat", "overwhelm", "defeat" and "hit", while the typical metaphor words for "Race" include "triumph", "win", "gain". Through comparison, we can find that in the eyes of BBC, "Success" can only be realized either through fighting or through fierce competition. In other words, BBC's understanding of "Success" is more like a zero-sum game, in which one can only achieve by defeating others or taking something away from others. That is why when we look at the main words under "Success" theme, all we can find are words that highlight "Fighting" and "Competition". The definition of "Success" from *China Daily* is depicted as a "growing tree", which does not harm or hurt others, but only uses the common resources the tree can have access to. Thus China's development will not pose any danger or threat to the surrounding countries, instead, a fruitful and growing tree can contribute to the ecological system. On the contrary, BBC News views "Success", China's success in particular, as the strengthening of an animated "power". The established scenario for international community is not a peaceful and balanced forest, where each tree has its own space for growth. Instead, the image constructed for international society by BBC is more like a "Dark forest", where all animated creature's only rule of living is through "fighting". The strongest animal will be the most successful one, and there is no other way that can lead to success. According to this logic, those who are becoming stronger and are eager to be successful can only reach their goal by "defeating" others. This is also the reason why the Western countries are so afraid of China's fast development. Moreover, their "China Threat" theory is also based on this logic. Because the Western countries deeply uphold such view of the world order, they naturally assume that along with China's development, China will definitely seek international hegemony and take away the privileges enjoyed by the developed countries. Yet as we can see from China's view on "Success", the seek for peace is deeply rooted in Chinese people's blood and its conceptualization of the world.

Instead of viewing the world as a "Dark forest" with all the countries as living creatures in the forest fighting for their lives, China sees the world as a harmonious forest with all the countries being the growing trees within this ecological system. As all the countries are "trees" that grow in the same land, the interests of all the "trees" are intertwined and what we need to do is to protect the environment together and co-build a brighter future for the "forest".

Now that we have compared the understanding of "Success" between *China Daily* and BBC News, *China Daily* represents China's view and BBC News stands for the perspective from the Western world. Through the comparison, we have a better understanding of how Chinese culture and the Western culture differ in their definitions and interpretations of success as well as the ways to achieve success. Apart from the "Success" theme, we also looked at words that belong to the "Failure" theme of BBC's reports to see if the understanding of "Failure" is consistent with the interpretation of "Success". As mentioned above, the representative words for the theme "Failure" include "lost", "on one's knees", "down the drain", "bungle" and "vain". Similarly, the top metaphor used in describing "Failure" is also the "Fight" or "War" metaphor. "Lost" is seen as the major failure. Besides, the ontological metaphor "Down is failure" is frequently used, as can be seen in phrases like "down the drain", "on one's knees", signifying that "going down" means failing. For example, "Their credibility is down the drain."

The last pair of contrast listed in Table 2-12 is between the verbal themes. As can be seen from Table 2-12, verbal themes like "Giving/Finding/Showing" have a relatively high ranking in contrast to the themes from BBC, which is featured by "Putting/Pulling/Pushing". Judging by the verbs themselves, there is hardly any specific metaphor that is involved. However, when we look at all the representative words of these two semantic themes, there emerges an overall personalized role. In the depiction of *China Daily*, Chinese government is a responsible "servant" and "guide" to the people, who is "giving" the people what they need, "finding" the people what they are looking for, and "showing" the people the road ahead. On the contrary, the constructed figure from BBC News is more like a "controller" or "manipulator", who is "putting" the people in places they do not want to be, and "pulling" or "pushing" them here and there. The main verbs included in the "Putting/Pulling/Pushing" theme are mostly causative verbs that are used in caused motion constructions that can lead to the physical movement of the patients. When those causative verbs are frequently used, it is very likely that the subject of the sentence will be constructed as an arbitrary and controlling figure who is used to imposing his or her own will on others.

In summary, the contrast in semantic themes between *China Daily* and BBC News reveals more metaphors used in constructing China's international image. Compared with BBC's entrenched stereotype of China, *China Daily* presents China with a more objective tone, as evidenced by the fact that there is not any "Evaluation: good" included in BBC's reports, while *China Daily* is featured by both "good" and "bad" evaluation. It is hard to say the Western media are adopting a neutral position towards China when their reports on China do not have any "good" evaluation at all. Another evidence to prove that *China Daily* is more objective is the number and type of "sensory" metaphors. As mentioned above, sensory metaphor belongs to ontological category. The adoption of sensory metaphor can appeal more to the reader's emotion, while at the same time reducing the objectivity of the accounted event. Especially when sensory metaphor is used not to share opinion but to report facts, the subjective glamour would be even more peculiar. In the reports from *China Daily*, very few sensory metaphors are spotted, while "Sensory: sight" metaphor is employed very frequently in BBC News. The frequent usage of the "Sight" metaphor not only increases the subjectivity of the accounting, but also contributes to distancing an abstract China image from the real China. The stress on "seeing" and "witnessing" results in an "onlooker" or "bystander" image of China which does not exist; and BBC News steps into this "imagined" China role to judge and evaluate what is happening in China, which gives the reader a fake sense that BBC is not making conclusion or judgement, and it is the imagined China who is discussing the matters in China.

2.4 Visualization of Key Metaphor Words in *China Daily* and BBC News

In this section, the key metaphors identified in the established corpus of *China*

Daily and BBC News are visualized using the word sketch function of Sketch Engine (Table 2-13). Typical words representing the key metaphors are analyzed and compared in terms of their frequent collocates. By doing so, we can gain a deeper understanding of the conceptualization of disease in Eastern and Western cultures, leading to the construction of a comprehensive semantic network in disease cognition between Chinese speakers and English speakers.

Table 2-13 Key metaphors and their representative keywords in *China Daily* and BBC News

Conceptual Metaphors	Searching Keywords
Fire metaphor	Spark
Spatial metaphor	Down/Up
Water metaphor	Flow
Journey metaphor	Step
Construction metaphor	Build
Plant metaphor	Grow
War metaphor	Fight
Sense metaphor	See
Game metaphor	Player

After searching the above keywords in the corpus of BBC's reports and *China Daily*'s reports, we have further proved which metaphor is more frequently used in which source, and what are the highlighted features of certain metaphors (Table 2-13). According to the searching results, the "Fire" metaphor is more frequently used in BBC, while the "Water" metaphor is favored in *China Daily*, as illustrated in the following figures.

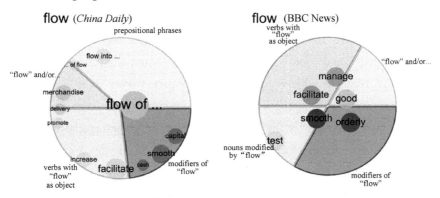

Figure 2-3 Word sketch of "flow" in *China Daily* and BBC News

It can be seen from the word sketch of "flow" in *China Daily* and BBC News that "flow" has more collocates in *China Daily*. The metaphorical word is used to describe the transportation of merchandise, capital and cash. Besides, verbs that co-occur with the word "flow" are more diversified, such as "increase", "promote", and "facilitate", while the word sketch of "flow" in BBC News enjoys fewer collocates. Given "flow" is a typical metaphorical word for the "Water" metaphor, we can conclude the "Water" metaphor is more common in *China Daily* than in BBC News.

The fact that the "Water" metaphor is preferred by *China Daily* is hardly surprising. "Water" has always been a favored image in Chinese culture. There are several reasons for the popularity of the "Water" metaphor in Chinese culture. Firstly, "water" presents itself as a less aggressive power, which is in line with the peaceful nature of Chinese culture. Secondly, water is closely associated with the image of "Junzi", which is the social model erected by Confucius. "Water" is frequently used to describe the personal relationship between "Junzi" for its purity and simplicity. The third reason goes to the modesty, tenacity, resilience, and inclusiveness of water. Those qualities of water overlap with the treasured merits in Chinese culture. Just like water, Chinese culture flows gently, but also continuously; and the characteristics of "Junzi" also resemble the features of water: pure, simple, modest, and persistent.

Although the "Water" metaphor featured by the word "flow" is not favored in BBC's accounts on China, the "Fire" metaphor does play an important role in the description of China's situation. As can be seen from Figure 2-4, the typical word that activates the "Fire" metaphor, the word "spark" enjoys much more collocates in BBC News compared with *China Daily* (Figure 2-4). In the word sketch of "spark" in BBC News, we can easily spot the two most frequent collocates, "death" and "fear", of which "death" is the subject of "spark", and "fear" is the frequent object of "spark". Apart from "fear", words like "outcry", "panic" and "anger" are listed as the objects of the verb "spark". The "Fire" metaphor activated by the word "spark" is highlighting the disorder and possible chaotic consequences caused by fire, and spread like fire too. The "Fire" metaphor triggered by the word "spark" is usually used to describe the fury and anger of people, creating a scene that the public is filled with anger. The "Fire" metaphor is used to exaggerate the negative emotion of the people, making the readers of the article feel that the outrageous Chinese people are about to develop a kind of "anger fire" capable of destroying and devouring everything! The application of the "Fire" metaphor in reporting some accidents and tragedies happened during the pandemic can magnify the anger and frustration of individuals who are involved in the events, and stir up the emotion of readers, preventing readers from seeing the bigger picture of what was happening in China.

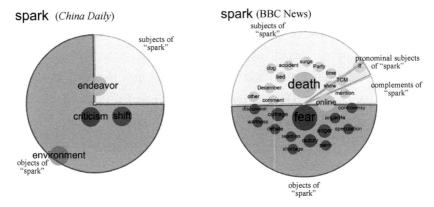

Figure 2-4 Word sketch of "spark" in *China Daily* and BBC News

China Daily uses more "Water" metaphors, while BBC News prefers "Fire" metaphors in their reports on China. But both sources employ a large number of "Journey" metaphors, albeit with different selection of metaphorical features. Take the word "step" as an example. We have generated the word sketches of both these two words, as shown in Figure 2-5.

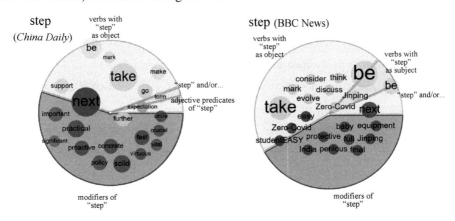

Figure 2-5 Word sketches of "step" in *China Daily* and BBC News

It can be seen from Figure 2-5 that the "verbs" with "step" as an object are more diversified in BBC's reports on China. Apart from the common verbs like "take", "make", "mark", BBC also uses verbs like "think", "consider" and "discuss". These verbs are "mental" verbs, that is, verbs used to describe the activities of mind rather than the body. What we can deduce from this point is that when it comes to the discussion of future path of China's development, BBC News, who usually steps into the shoes of that distanced abstract China, would like to present China as less decisive and hesitant in choosing which step to take. The suspicion of the path for development does not exist in *China Daily*'s reports, the main verbs that have "steps" as objects are action verbs with strong agency, demonstrating the determination and decisiveness of China in taking its solid steps in the road of development. The differences in highlighted features of the "Journey" metaphor can also be reflected in the adjectives used to modify "step". The modifiers for "step" from *China Daily* are mainly adjectives with positive semantic prosody, such as "significant", "concrete", "proactive", "virtuous", "vital", "practical", while the modifiers before "step" in BBC are not. There are much fewer modifiers for "step" in BBC News, and some of them are questioning or criticizing the "step" taken, for example, "baby", "perilous", and "protective", all of which are not in favor of the steps taken. In fact, Western media like BBC News have no rights to smear China just because China is not doing the same as them, and their arrogant judgement of China's measures in fighting the pandemic is also under the influence of their bias. That is why coronavirus has become the most politicized virus in human civilization. BBC's lashing out at China's Covid-prevention measures is a reflection of their anger that China is walking on a different path successfully and their fear that China will become stronger than them, which in their world will inevitably lead to the seek for hegemony.

Another prominent metaphor in *China Daily* is the "Construction" metaphor, of which the construction of buildings is the source domain, and the development of abstract concept is usually the target domain. The typical word used in the "Construction" metaphor is "build". Using "build" as the keyword, we have generated the word sketch of "build" in both *China Daily* and BBC News (Figure 2-6). The comparison of the two word sketches can unveil more differences and similarities in the value and attitudes between East and West.

Chapter 2 Corpus-Based Comparison of Disease Metaphors in English and Chinese

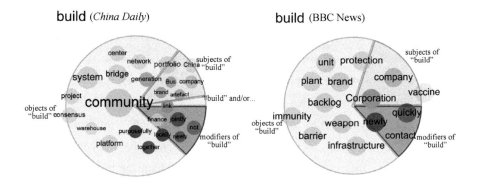

Figure 2-6   Word sketches of "build" in *China Daily* and BBC News

As shown in Figure 2-6, the top collocate for "build" in *China Daily* is the word "community". That is to say, the "Construction" metaphor is mainly used to illustrate China's willingness to further the development of community. Given the reports are collected from *China Daily*, here the "community" China is so eager to "build" is not the local community, but rather the international community with all friendly countries in the world. Consistent with the popularity of the "Water" metaphor, the vision of a prosper and stronger China is not aggressive and will not pose any threat to other countries. China believes that a peaceful and harmonious international community is the ideal environment for win-win and common prosperity. The "community" will not be "built" by China alone. As can be seen from the modifiers of "build", China wants to "build" the community "jointly", "together" with other countries. Besides, other objects like "consensus", "platform", and "bridge" are all explaining what Chinese want to say to the world using the "Construction" metaphor. Simply put, it would be a invitation to build the world a better place together. Different from the "Construction" metaphor used in *China Daily*, the word sketch of the word "build" in BBC presents us a less promising future. Instead of using "build" metaphorically, we can see from Figure 2-6 that most of the "objects" of the verb "build" are actual things rather than abstract concepts. For example, we have "weapon", "plant", "infrastructure", all of which are common objects of "build". Within the limited objects of the verb "build", we can identify several words that can count as "Construction" metaphors, such as "protection", "immunity" and "barrier" in certain contexts. The focus of BBC's report on China

97

adopts a micro perspective, instead of looking at the long-term development of mankind, BBC's report only focuses on the short-term effect of the measures taken to curb the virus. The fact that *China Daily* and BBC have clear different focuses in using the "Construction" metaphor reflects the default perspective of China and the West. Represented by *China Daily*, China is used to look at the big picture and make long-term plan, such as the construction of community with shared future for mankind. On the contrary, Western media like BBC stand for the conventionalized view of the West, that is to grab on what is in one's hand and is more concerned with the current issue.

Besides "Construction" metaphor, the "Plant" metaphor is more explicit in *China Daily*'s reports. As can be seen in Table 2-12 of this chapter, there are quite a few plant-related metaphors, including "flourish", "thrive" and "fruitful", all of which are not found in BBC News. But we can also find the "Plant" metaphor in the accounts from BBC News, only in a more implicit way. For example, the word "grow" is only etymologically used to refer to the maturation of plants rather than animals or human beings. The root from its Proto-Indo-European form "ghre" means to grow, and become green. Thus we understand that the meaning of the word "grow" expands through metaphor, by projecting the "growing" of plants to the "growing" of humans and other animals. Although the meaning of "grow" has become conventionalized nowadays, which includes the maturation of all creatures, the use of this word still triggers some semantic association with the growing of plants. We believe that this lingering association with "growing plant" is stronger with Chinese character 长 (grow) due to the hieroglyphic nature of Chinese language. This may also be one of the reasons why the "Plant" metaphor is more common and explicit both in *China Daily*'s reports and in Chinese language in general. Now let us take a look at the word sketches of "grow" in the corpus of *China Daily* and that of BBC News in Figure 2-7.

Chapter 2 Corpus-Based Comparison of Disease Metaphors in English and Chinese

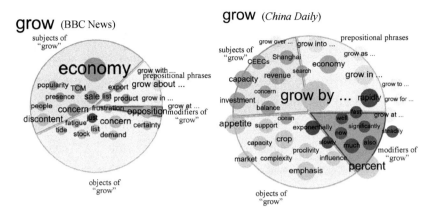

Figure 2-7 Word sketches of "grow" in *China Daily* and BBC News

At first sight, we can notice from Figure 2-7 that the number of collocates of "grow" in *China Daily* is more than that in BBC News (on the left). Taking a further look at both word sketches, we can find that there are very few "modifiers" in BBC News for "grow", the only modifier that is shown in the above figure is "just", which usually indicates that the "grow" is limited. However, from *China Daily*, we can find much more modifiers, including "exponentially", "much", "significantly", "fast" and "steadily". The majority of the modifiers for the word "grow" is stressing the fast speed or large extent of growth. It is justified to say that *China Daily*, as an official English journal of China, may intend to use more positive modifiers to demonstrate China's achievement to the world. But we can also spot modifiers like "slowly" from *China Daily*, meaning that the reports not solely focus on the positive side, but also stick to the facts when the "growth" is indeed "slow". The inclusion of both "positive" and "negative" modifiers serve as a demonstration of *China Daily*'s more objective attitude in accounting for what happened in China. Besides, we can spot the same tendency in the objects and subjects of the word "grow", the objects and subjects of "grow" include words of different semantic prosodies. For example, we can see words like "capacity", "support", we can also notice relatively negative words such as "complexity" and "proclivity", and there are neutral words like "market", "influence" and "emphasis". The frequency (indicated by the size of the circle) of these words is similar too. However, the objects of "grow" from BBC News are not evenly distributed, the words that caught our eyes from the word sketch are "concern", "opposition"; there are words like "fatigue", "frustration"; and there are hardly any words with a definite positive prosody, albeit we do see neutral words like "certainty", "demand", "stock", which are used less frequently. Within the subjects for "grow", we can find in BBC News the predominant word is "economy", and all the other words like "discontent", "concern" are used less frequently. To the opposite, the subjects for "grow" in *China Daily* are evenly distributed, not only "economy" can grow, "revenue", "capacity" and "investment" can "grow" too. Besides, it is also worth noting that the most frequent prepositional phrase from *China Daily* is "grow by", and the preposition "by" is often followed by the extent of growth, which suggests that more attention is paid to the "fruit" of growth. The same result-oriented cognition can also be seen in the prepositional phrase "grow into". However, the prepositional phrase included in the word sketch of "grow" in BBC News is paying less attention to the "outcome", as can be seen from the phrases like "grow with", "grow in", "grow at", "grow about". Attention is paid more to the process of the growing rather than the outcome. The "Plant" metaphor includes more than the word "grow". We will discuss more about the "Plant" metaphor through the discussion of words like "root" in the following sections.

The remaining three pairs of metaphors are "War" metaphor, "Sense" metaphor and "Game" metaphor. The word we chose to stand for "War" metaphor is the word "fight", and we searched for the collocates of "fight" in the corpus of *China Daily* and that of BBC News. The top 5 collocates of "fight" in these two sources are shown in the following tables.

Table 2-14 Top 5 collocates of the word "fight" in *China Daily*

Words	Cooccurrences	Candidates	T-score	MI	LogDice
against	16	108	4.00	9.94	11.89
supplied	4	6	2.00	12.11	11.83
pandemic	13	182	3.60	8.89	10.97
disease	4	38	2.00	9.45	10.91
COVID-19	14	233	3.73	8.64	10.77

Chapter 2 Corpus-Based Comparison of Disease Metaphors in English and Chinese

Table 2-15 Top 5 collocates of the word "fight" in BBC News

Words	Cooccurrences	Candidates	T-score	MI	LogDice
painful	6	10	2.45	11.33	12.03
against	8	124	2.82	8.11	10.67
year	8	204	2.81	7.39	10.09
pandemic	3	121	1.72	6.73	9.28
virus	7	393	2.61	6.25	9.06

From the above two tables, we can learn that the object of "fight" is usually the pandemic, disease, virus or Covid-19 in the reports on China from both *China Daily* and BBC News. However, the top-ranking word in Table 2-15 is "painful", which highlights the difficult fighting process and implicates the damage and sacrifice made during the fight. On the contrary, the distinctive collocate of "fight" in *China Daily* is "supplied", and the common context is like "The country also dispatched 38 expert teams to 34 countries to help them fight the disease and supplied over 2.2 billion vaccines to more than 120 countries and international organizations." The verb "supply" co-occurs with "fight" to increase the chance of "winning". The cognitive effect of the co-occurrence of these two verbs is that the readers' attention will be drawn mainly to the results of the fight rather than the process. The difference in the feature selection of the "Fight" metaphor reflects the similar cognitive traits between English and Chinese. As mentioned above, during the discussion of the "Plant" metaphor, Chinese language, represented by *China Daily*, pays more attention to the results of the action; however, English language, represented by BBC News, attaches more importance to the "process" of the action.

About the "Sense" metaphor, we have learned that BBC News is featured by the "Sight" metaphor, which personifies "China" as an individual who passively "witnesses" what happened in China. Yet in the previous texts, we have not investigated the "Sight" metaphor in *China Daily* and how it is different from the description in BBC News. We will first compare the word sketches of "see" in both corpora in Figure 2-8.

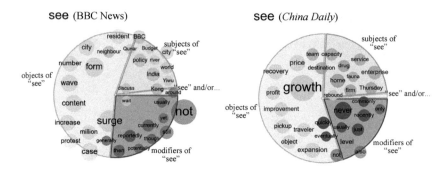

Figure 2-8　Word sketches of "see" in *China Daily* and *BBC News*

From Figure 2-8 we can learn that both *China Daily* and *BBC News* use plenty of "Sight" metaphors, yet what China "sees" is very different from that "seen" by BBC. From the word sketch of "see" in *BBC News*, we can find that the most frequent object is "surge", given that the reports are about China's situation during the pandemic, we can deduce that the "surge" here probably refers to the sharp increase of cases. For example, "China is currently seeing a surge in Covid cases, with reports of hospitals and crematorium being overwhelmed". Differently, the most frequent collocate for "see" in the reports from *China Daily* is "growth", the common context of which is like "… might see a relatively strong growth in exports with effective vaccine immunization in many countries". This clear contrast in the frequent collocates for the verb "see" between "surge" and "growth" is that "growth" is usually the expected results while "surge" indicates something unexpected and often undesirable. Therefore, in terms of the same "Sight" metaphor, we can reveal various emphasis on the things that the two sides would like to pay attention to.

　　The last metaphorical category is the "Game" metaphor. As discussed above, "player" is hardly used metaphorically in BBC's reports on China. The "Game" metaphor usually takes the form of the "Race" metaphor in *BBC News*, and "Race" can also be categorized as a kind of "Game". Thus we use two different keywords to search the corpora of *China Daily* and *BBC News* respectively. For the "Game" metaphor in *China Daily*, we use "player" as the keyword and deliver the word sketch for "player". For the "Race" metaphor in *BBC News*, we use "beat" as the searching word and generated the word sketch for "beat". Although the searching words are not the same, the results can demonstrate the overall view towards "Game" from the two sources (Figure 2-9).

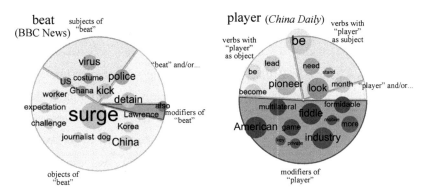

Figure 2-9 Word sketches of "beat" in BBC News and "player" in *China Daily*

The search of "beat" has only three records in *China Daily*, and only two of them are using "beat" metaphorically. For example, "Chinese Internet heavyweight Tencent posted an 11 percent rise in revenue within the first quarter, beating analyst expectations and showcasing a sound growth momentum." Another context is "More people are taking to hiking in the mountains or setting up campsites this summer, as they seek to stay healthy, beat everyday stress and foster ecological awareness." Among these two example sentences, the first "beat" triggers the "Race" metaphor, as in Tencent's rise overtakes the expectations of analyst. The second "beat" does not activate the "Race" metaphor, but rather triggers the "Fight" metaphor, as if "everyday stress" is the enemy. Similarly, despite that there are plenty of "Player" metaphors in *China Daily*, we only find three records of "Player" in BBC's reports on China. For example, "A lot of the players have already diversified some of their resources and their plans, not to put all their eggs in one basket" and "All players and staff at the tournament must be vaccinated or have an exemption granted by an expert independent panel." Only in these two sentences, "player" triggers the "Game" metaphor as if the enterprises are all "players" in a "game" of money making.

As can be seen from the word sketch of "beat" in BBC News (Figure 2-9), "Surge" is believed to be the major enemy, and the runner-up frequent object of "beat" is "China", while the main subjects of "beat" include "virus", "police" and "US". The frequent subjects and objects of "beat" can reflect how BBC News uses the "Race" metaphor, that is, what kind of "Race" is usually activated. Two main kinds of "Race" can be revealed. One is the "Race" between the US and China. In the description of BBC, China is usually placed as the object of "beat", suggesting that US is taking the lead. The second "Race" is between "virus" and China, in which China is still placed in the position of "object", indicating that China is more likely to lose the battle against the virus. In both kinds, the focus is laid on the results of a competition—one can either win or lose, beat others or be beaten, which is in line with the zero-sum Cold War mindset of the West world.

From the word sketch of "player" in Figure 2-9, we can have a better understanding of what fields are the domains that can be compared to the "playground" for the "players" to play. As can be seen from the modifiers of "player", we see words like "industry" and "multilateral", from which we can see that the "playground" can cover both "economic" and "political" fields; and the frequent use of "multilateral" reflects China's emphasis on the multi-polarization tendency in the international stage. The words "American" and "fiddle" are the frequent modifiers of "player", but these two words are not used to modifier "player" as a metaphorical word.

In summary, the metaphors we identified in the reports on China's Covid prevention activities share both similarities and differences. Similar metaphors that exist in both reports include "Journey" metaphor, "Plant" metaphor, and "War" metaphor. Although the two sources share these metaphors in common, *China Daily* and *BBC News* differ in the selection of more specific metaphorical features. Apart from the metaphors that the two media share in common, there are metaphors that only exist in either *China Daily* or *BBC News*. For example, there are a few "Fire" metaphors in BBC News, which can not be found in *China Daily*; on the contrary, *China Daily* is featured by a lot of "Water" metaphors, while BBC News is not. Moreover, the "Construction" metaphor is one of the essential conceptual metaphors used in *China Daily*, while there is very few this kind of metaphor in BBC News.

Another major metaphor that exists in both sources is the "Space" metaphor. The representative words of the "Space" metaphor are "up" and "down", but *China Daily* and *BBC News* differ in the percentage of using "up" or "down". By searching for both "up" and "down", we found the ratio of the number of collocates for "up" and "down" in BBC News is $69/79 = 0.87$, while the ratio in

China Daily is 108/12 = 9. The ratio between "up" and "down" indicates that in terms of "Space" metaphor, *China Daily* lays predominate emphasis on the "up" direction, while BBC News attaches relatively equal importance to both "up" and "down".

Table 2-16 Top 10 collocates for "up" in both *China Daily* and BBC News

Sources	No.	Words	Cooccurrences	Candidates	T-Score	MI	LogDice
BBC News	1	filling	14	14	3.74	9.49	10.93
	2	set	15	53	3.85	7.67	10.81
	3	opening	9	17	2.99	8.57	10.28
	4	signing	6	6	2.45	9.49	9.76
	5	ramping	6	6	2.45	9.49	9.76
	6	step	6	24	2.44	7.49	9.65
	7	picked	5	5	2.23	9.49	9.50
	8	opened	5	11	2.23	8.35	9.46
	9	surveillance	5	22	2.22	7.35	9.40
	10	held	5	30	2.22	6.90	9.35
China Daily	1	set	37	77	6.07	8.42	11.73
	2	percent	65	508	7.97	6.52	11.40
	3	year-on-year	25	123	4.97	7.18	10.99
	4	efforts	16	149	3.95	6.26	10.26
	5	step	11	34	3.30	7.85	10.17
	6	shore	10	10	3.16	9.48	10.15
	7	speed	8	17	2.82	8.39	9.79
	8	first	14	345	3.61	4.86	9.52
	9	making	7	44	2.62	6.83	9.47
	10	percentage	7	44	2.62	6.83	9.47

It can be seen from Table 2-16 that in most cases, "up" follows another verb, such as "step up", "speed up", "open up", "pick up". Apart from being part of the fixed phrase, the frequent collocate for "up" is "surveillance", while the frequent words that collocate with "up" are "percent", "efforts", "making" and "percentage". Take "efforts" as an example. It is one of the frequent objects of phrasal verbs that contain "up", such as "ramp up efforts to build modern logistics infrastructure networks", "ratchet up efforts to help companies resume operations in regions hit hard by the pandemic", "stepped up efforts to localize its business in the country". From these concrete examples, we can learn that "efforts" is the common target domain for space in *China Daily*. "Efforts" are made more concrete through "spatial conceptualization", as if the "efforts" are something that can be piled together and when more "efforts" are made, the pile becomes higher.

Table 2-17 Top 10 collocates for "down" in both *China Daily* and BBC News

Sources	No.	Words	Cooccurrences	Candidates	T-Score	MI	LogDice
BBC News	1	locked	41	49	6.40	9.75	12.69
	2	step	8	24	2.82	8.42	10.52
	3	shut	7	28	2.64	8.01	10.30
	4	authorities	8	141	2.78	5.87	9.80
	5	stand	4	8	2.00	9.01	9.66
	6	district	4	22	1.99	7.55	9.54
	7	come	5	79	2.20	6.03	9.46
	8	area	4	33	1.98	6.96	9.45
	9	small	4	36	1.98	6.84	9.43
	10	communities	3	10	1.73	8.27	9.23
China Daily	1	percentage	8	44	2.83	10.24	11.79
	2	point	6	38	2.45	10.04	11.50
	3	April	6	114	2.44	8.45	10.42
	4	quarter	3	121	1.72	7.36	9.35
	5	first	3	345	1.70	5.85	8.03
	6	percent	4	508	1.96	5.71	7.93
	7	this	3	397	1.70	5.65	7.85
	8	Chinese	3	575	1.68	5.12	7.34
	9	from	4	778	1.94	5.10	7.34
	10	on	3	1253	1.62	3.99	6.26

In the corpus of *China Daily*, the word "down" appeared only 20 times, enjoying merely 12 frequent collocates. "Down" is often used as an adverb in *China Daily*, which is used to describe the specific percentage that is reduced. For example, "the purchasing managers" index for China's manufacturing sector came

Chapter 2　Corpus-Based Comparison of Disease Metaphors in English and Chinese

in at 47.4 in April, down from 49.5 in March, "the sub-index for production stood at 44.4 in April, down 5.1 percentage points from the reading in March". Very rarely is "down" used in a verbal phrase, such as "crack down", for example, "the United States to crack down on Chinese technology products and apps such as TikTok". To the opposite, quite a few of the collocates for "down" in BBC News are verbs, and with "down", the verbal phrase is completed. For example, "lock down", "step down", "stand down". Through the comparison, we can learn that "down", as a keyword for the "Space" metaphor, is more frequently used to depict a macro and abstract phenomenon or trend in BBC News, while "down" is used with a much less degree of metaphoricity in *China Daily*, referring to the decrease of certain value. In summary, the way that "down" is used in BBC News resembles the way "up" is employed in *China Daily*.

The clear contrast in the use of the "Space" metaphor can also be reflected in the application of the "Plant" metaphor, especially metaphors based on more fundamental part of the plant—"root". In fact, many disease metaphors in both English and Chinese include metaphors that take "root" as a source domain. We will focus on the comparison between disease metaphors with English "root" and Chinese 根 in the next chapter.

In this chapter, we intend to demonstrate the differences in space-time cognition by contrasting the English translations of Chinese "Plant" metaphors composed by English and Chinese translators. The materials used for analysis are two English versions of the classic Chinese novel *Dream of the Red Mansion* translated by David Hawks and Yang Xianyi. We first hypothesize that Chinese is more space-oriented in plant conceptualization, while English is more time-oriented. We analyzed the cognitive reasons behind different translation strategies adopted for the same "Plant" metaphor and verified the deduction from example analysis in the corpus. The typical "Plant" metaphor analyzed in the research is the "Root" metaphor. The results indicate that most Chinese "Root" metaphors are "double-imaged" metonymic metaphors, which rely on the hierarchical correlation between plant components and the accumulation of spacial characteristics through multiple metonymies embedded in metaphorical projection. On the contrary, the conceptualization of "root" and "plant" in English pay more attention to the dynamic growth of the plant rather than the spacial relations between different parts.

Cognitive and Contrastive Analysis of Disease Metaphors in English and Chinese

Chapter 3

Spatial-Temporal Cognition Analysis of Disease Metaphors in English and Chinese

The conceptualization of space and time in different languages has always been a hot topic for scholars and researchers in cognitive linguistics. Since Lakoff & Johnson (1980) demonstrated the influence of language on cognition through the illustration of conceptual metaphors, researchers began to pay more attention to the conceptualizing or cognitive differences between languages and their influence on thinking. Langacker argued that our brain "construe" situations and images during language comprehension, which highlights spacial concepts in our conceptualization of the world (Langacker, 1987, 2013). Besides, many other scholars analyzed spatial-temporal metaphors to reveal the cognitive commonness and varieties in space-time cognition (Grady, 1997; Kovecses, 2005). Meanwhile, many Chinese scholars, especially those interested in the cognitive comparison between English and Chinese, have devoted themselves to the space-time cognition contrast between English and Chinese (Wang, 2013). Recent studies are arguing that there is a dichotomy between time and space in English due to the significant variance in the "entrance" of verbs and nouns in English sentence composition, while time and space are conflated in Chinese, drawing evidence from the inner structure of Chinese characters, as well as grammars (Liu & Xu, 2019). However, most of the previous studies about space and time have taken the macro semantic approach and are limited to analytical studies with limited support from the corpus. Very few have attempted to reflect the cross-cultural cognitive differences through the comparative analysis of translation strategies with statistical evidence from the corpus (Hu, 2011).

Based on human's familarity of plant growing, root is commonly used metaphorically to better understand the world around us. As an essential part of

Chapter 3 Spatial-Temporal Cognition Analysis of Disease Metaphors in English and Chinese

plant, "root" encompasses several basic meanings both in Chinese ard English, such as [underground] [source of nutrition], etc. One of the main root metaphors is "root as the cause of disease".

This chapter hypothesizes that Chinese is more space-oriented while English is more time-oriented in the cognition of "root = cause of disease", and aims to prove the hypothesis by analyzing the "root = cause of disease" metaphor translations (E-C) given by two translators, who are native speakers of English and Chinese. The distinguishing features in the metaphor formation and interpretation support the hypothesis that the reason for choosing different translating strategies adopted by the two translators can be attributed to their accustomed schematization of plants, of which Chinese relies more on the hierarchical spacial construction of plant components, while English translator's cognition depends more on the temporal changes of a plant's spatial characteristics as a whole.

We first compared the translations for "root = cause of disease" metaphors, and then analyzed the cognitive reasons behind the translation strategies. Examples are from the two English translation versions of the classic Chinese novel—*A Dream of Red Mansions*. "Root" is used as the keyword for corpus searching, and we carried out statistical analysis of the retrieved material to further prove the differences in space-time cognition between English and Chinese in terms of disease cognition.

3.1 Different Disease Metaphors with "Root" in English and 根 in Chinese

According to Talmy (2000), our conceptualization of space involves two systems: One system is the frame to load things or locate things, and the other is the content of frame, including the shapes and relationships of the content. And there are three types of relations between the content with spatial features and the spatial framework. The first is the spatial characteristics of an object itself; the second is the relative spatial location between different objects; the third is the spatial correlation between the components of an object, including a potential "schemata" and the "arrangement" between its components. The categorization provides a clear framework to understand which type of spatial relation is highlighted in plant conceptualization between English and Chinese.

Besides, the study of "attention", which is rooted in psychology, is brought into the cognitive study of languages (Shu, 2008). That is, language can place the focus of attention on some components of a situation by directly mentioning the features, while placing the other components in the background. The cognitive process associated with this phenomenon is called "windowing of attention", of which the referred situation is called "event frame". What's placed into the spot is the "window", while the parts being backgrounded are called "gap" (Talmy, 2000). In this book, "windowing of attention" is used as a theoretical approach in analyzing the cognitive process behind the choice of translations for "Plant" metaphors. We hypothesize that the "windowing of attention" varies between English and Chinese plant conceptualization, spatial features of the plant are those being "windowed" in Chinese while those in the "window" are temporal changes of the spatial features of the plant in English, which provides evidence to the hypothetical space-time cognition contrast between the two languages.

The space-cognition contrast in disease or problem between English and Chinese can be demonstrated in the following "Root" metaphor translations.

a. 方剪草除根,保住自己的名誉。(第六十九回,第172页)

(Literal translation: Cut the grasses and remove the root, so can you save your reputation.)

a1. Only by such root-and-branch methods, she felt, could her fears be allayed and the threat to her reputation be removed. (Hawkes, Chapter 69, p.1363)

a2. In this way the root of the trouble would be removed and her reputation assured. (Yang, Chapter 69, p.1238)

Yang's translation is closer to the conventional meaning of the Chinese four-character phrase 剪草除根, in which 根(root) is considered the most essential part of the grass compared with other components, therefore the attention focus of the Chinese fixed phrase 剪草除根 (剪 = cut, 草 = grass, 除 = remove, 根 = root) is on the second part—除根 (remove the root), which emphasizes the hierarchical spatial structure between the components of a plant. Similarly, the cognition of a problem in Chinese also resembles the static configuration of a plant, in which root is considered as the fundamental layer of the problem, thus the elimination of root would solve the problem once and for all. However, 剪草 and 除根 share equal syntactical status, the trivial difference has to be perceived by semantic analysis, and the semantic analysis is restrained by the schemata in plant conceptualization in different languages and cultures.

As a native Chinese speaker, we can assume that Yang possesses the Chinese schemata in Chinese root conceptualization, and from Yang's translation choice, our assumption can be partially verified. Yang did not translate the phrase literally as "to cut the grass and remove the root". Instead, he adapted the English form to maintain the essence of the phrase by translating it simply into "the root of the trouble would be removed", omitting the "grass-cutting". On the contrary, Hawks's translation of "root-and-branch methods" reserved the syntactical format of the original phrase. Besides, "root-and-branch methods" is also a conventional English phrase, emphasizing the resoluteness of doing something.

However, different from "windowing" the importance of "root" as an essential component in a plant as a whole, Hawks's translation demonstrates that he perceives the most resolute way to eliminate a plant is to curb its growing process in a "root-and-branch" way, of which "root" stands for the downward growth, while "branch" represents the upward growth. Hawks's emphasis in the spatial cognition of grass is on the physical characteristics of grass, which is made of the branches above the ground and the underground root rather than the hierarchical relationship between different components. The individual spatial characteristics of the grass as unity are "windowed" against a time-oriented schema, the most logical way to "remove the grass = solve the problem" is to wipe the problem out in a "root-and-branch way".

The different translations of the same "Grass" metaphor demonstrate the disparity in space cognition between English and Chinese. In the process of using root to conceptualize diseases or problems, Yang puts more emphasis on the hierarchical relationship between the components of the disease/problem and the role each component plays in the whole framework, which is the third kind of spatial relationship that's being underscored (Talmy, 2008). Meanwhile, Hawks's cognition of the disease/problem relies on individualistic spatial characteristics, which is the first kind of spatial cognition according to Talmy's categorization. The

Cognitive and Contrastive Analysis of Disease Metaphors in English and Chinese

first type of space cognition is relatively more flexible and dynamic, which can be seen as the time-oriented space cognition.

From the above example analysis, we have reached a preliminary conclusion that the conceptualization of disease or problem in Chinese is relatively more static, relying mainly on space-oriented cognition, while English's conceptualization of disease/problem is more frequently intertwined with temporal concepts, which took the form of an "Event Framework" involving more actions represented in verbal forms.

"Subject + complement" is a very common Chinese sentence structure, and the usual correspondent English translation has to be "subject + be verb + complement". For example,

Chinese: (S) 天气 Weather　　(C) 很好 good
English: (S) Weather (be verb) is　　(C) good.

The time-oriented dynamic conceptualization of root in English is also found in Hawks's translation of the following sentence in *A Dream of Red Mansions*.

b. 薛家根基不错，且现今大富，薛蝌生得又好，且贾母又作保山。(第 57 回，第 412 页)

(Xue's have a fairly good root, and now they are very wealthy; Xue Ke is very handsome, and Grandmother Jia will be the match-maker.)

b1. Since the Xue's came of fairly good stock and were now very wealthy, while Xue Ke was a handsome young man, and the go-between, moreover, was no less a person than the Lady Dowager. (Yang, Chapter 57, p.579)

b2. The Xue family were of respectable origins; they were immensely rich; Xue Ke was a good-looking boy; and Grandmother Jia was making herself responsible for the match. (Hawkes, Chapter 57, p.614)

Hawks's translation of sentence b "were of respectable origins" falls into the same pattern of translation by adding the "be" verb between the subject and the adjective. It's argued by Langacker (1987) that compared with "be" verb, action verbs are more of a dynamic temporal concept. Now when we take a look at Yang's translation of sentence b "Xues came of fairly good stock", we can find that Yang used an action verb "came" instead of the "be" verb by default to

Chapter 3 Spatial-Temporal Cognition Analysis of Disease Metaphors in English and Chinese

compensate for the extra cognitive efforts required from the English readers to connect "fairly good stock" with a "good wealthy family background". Yang's translation can bridge the Chinese and English plant conceptualization differences, besides, it also implies that Chinese is more space-oriented while it's easier for English readers to deal with dynamic time-oriented concepts.

There's no denying that there is an overlapping between space-oriented cognition and time-oriented cognition since most matters can be understood and analyzed both as static objects and as developing events, and everything exists in space and time simultaneously. The difference lies in which is the dominant cognitive domain. In the conceptual root metaphor, the literal translation of the Chinese description 根基不错 is 根 = root, 基 = foundation, 不错 = fairly good. It can be found that more emphasis was placed on the stability of the hierarchical family structure by connecting "root" with "foundation". However, if the English translation of the phrase is composed as "Xue's have a fairly good root and foundation", it probably will confuse most of the English readers since their perception of the metaphor FAMILY IS A PLANT relies on the similarity of developing and growing process between the family and the plant rather than the stable constructional relationship between the components. Instead of vertical spacial growth, the image schema of a family is formed along the horizontal axis with stresses on involvement; therefore, the only logical way to understand the metaphor is by relating "root" to the "origin" of the family from a temporal perspective, and that's exactly what Hawks has chosen to do in translating the sentence as "The Xue family were of respectable origins."

It can be concluded from the above analysis that when the "double-imaged" "Plant" metaphor integrates plant and building, an image which enhances the hierarchical conceptualization of the plant, it's difficult for the metaphor to be understood by English readers. Yet there are also root metaphors that are maintained in both the English translations, examples can be found in the translation strategies adopted by Hawks and Yang in translating the plant metaphor—"root of illness".

c. 林丫头若不是这个病呢,我凭着花多少钱都使得。(第97回,第105页)

c1. If that's not the root of her illness, I'm willing to spend any sum to cure

Cognitive and Contrastive Analysis of Disease Metaphors in English and Chinese

her. (Hawkes, Chapter 97, p. 1050)

  d. 贾母等知他病未除根,不许他胡思乱想……(第98回,第1068页)

  d1. Knowing that the cause of his illness was not yet uprooted, his grandmother … (Yang, Chapter 98, p. 1068)

  From the translation of sentences c and d, we learned that both Hawks and Yang reserved the conceptual metaphor "Root as the Cause of Illness". One of the reasons for a more equivalent translation in form is that the spatial and temporal cognition of disease as a plant overlaps. Therefore, the cognitive efforts required to understand this metaphor are more or less the same even though the conceptualization of plant is more space-oriented in Chinese and more time-oriented in English.

  However, whether the Chinese "Plant" metaphor can be perceived easily by English readers depends on the other image integrated into the "double imaged" metaphor. The "Disease root" metaphor is reserved in Sentences c and d because disease is a concept that pays more or less equal attention to space and time in both English and Chinese. For other Chinese "Plant" metaphors, it's not easy for English readers who rely more on time-oriented plant conceptualization to comprehend. For example, the commonly accepted Chinese conceptual metaphor LIFE IS PLANT.

  e. 贾母咳道:"这是宝玉的命根子,因丢了,所以他这么失魂丧魄的。"(第95回,第669页)

  e1. "This jade is the root of Baoyu's life," sighed the old lady. "It's because he's lost it that he's out of his mind." (Yang, Chapter 95, p. 1036)

  e2. "The jade is Bao-yu's very life. Losing it is what has made him lose his wits." (Hawkes, Chapter 95, p. 981)

  The conceptual metaphor LIFE IS PLANT in Chinese is also a "double-imaged" metonymic metaphor based on the physiological similarity between a standing person and a vertical tree, which is a space-oriented conceptualization. Besides, because a plant is perceived as a hierarchical structure between different components with "root" as the baseline (Langacker, 2013) when the image schema of a plant projects onto human life, the Chinese metaphor 命根子 (the root of life, 命 = life, 根子 = root) is used to emphasize the importance of jade. The same metaphor is translated differently by Hawks and Yang. Yang's translation

Chapter 3   Spatial-Temporal Cognition Analysis of Disease Metaphors in English and Chinese

reserved the metaphor by literally translating it as "the root of Baoyu's life" because Yang, as a native Chinese speaker, subconsciously understands the metaphor between life and plant from a spacial perspective and is aware of the hierarchical relationship between the plant and components, therefore choose to reserve the metaphorical form. On the contrary, Hawks only translated the sentence as "The jade is Bao-yu's very life", omitting the "Plant" metaphor. The reason for his translation choice goes to the cognitive discrepancy between plant and conceptualization. It is the growing process of a plant that is highlighted in the conceptualization, thus when the English readers try to understand the metaphorical projection between life and plant, their dynamic developing features are focalized instead of the static comparison between the physiological appearance. Therefore, Hawks chose to focus on the meaning and translate the sentence as "The jade is Bao-yu's very life" to avoid possible misunderstanding, for the literal translation stands the risk that English readers might think that "the root of life" means that "Baoyu originates from the jade", which is quite different from the intended meaning of the original text.

From the above analysis of root-based disease metaphor translation, we can see that the translations adopted by English and Chinese translators are under the influence of their conceptualization of disease, or more specifically, the variance in the strategies used for root-based disease metaphor translation is in line with the gap between the cognitive efforts paid to the spacial concept between English and Chinese. When the gap is large, in other words, when the space-oriented cognition is the dominant domain in the root-based disease metaphor, it's more unlikely for the metaphor to be reserved by a native English translator. Examples include FAMILY IS PLANT and LIFE IS PLANT. On the contrary, when the gap is small, the formation of the disease metaphor requires similar cognitive efforts from space and time, in this condition the metaphor is more likely to be reserved in C-E translation in both two versions of translation. The translating strategies adopted by Yang and Hawks for the same root-based disease metaphor further proved the spacial-temporal contrast in cognition. At least when it comes to the conceptualization of plants, we can conclude that the cognition of plants in Chinese is more space-oriented, while that in English is more time-oriented. Moreover, when the space-oriented cognition is in the dominant position, usually more focus would be laid on the hierarchical structure and inter-relationship between various components of the matter. Meanwhile, when the time-oriented cognition is highlighted, more attention would be paid to the historical development and distinguishing features of the matter as a whole.

3.2 Corpus-Based Analysis of Disease Metaphors with Chinese 根 and English "Root"

Despite the analysis of typical root-based disease metaphor translations from *A Dream of Red Mansions*, the spacial-temporal contrast in plant conceptualization is further proved with statistical support from corpus search and the analysis of "root" related expressions in both English and Chinese. The data used in the following are drawn from Modern Chinese Corpus and COCA. 12,338 search results were found when we ran a search for the character 根 in the online corpus of Contemporary Chinese, 2,000 sentences were selected randomly as the material for further analysis. By running manual filtering of the 2,000 sentences, only 345 "Root" metaphors are found. Meanwhile, we have searched for the word "root" in the online corpus COCA and the first thousand sentences are chosen for analysis. Also by filtering the proper nouns and the other unqualified items, 372 "Root" metaphors are found.

Table 3-1 The proportion of specific "Root" metaphors in Chinese and English

No.	"Root" metaphor categorization (based on mearing)	Chinese 根 Metaphor (No./%)	English "Root" Metaphor (No./%)
1.	cause	根源(the cause of …) (153/32.6%)	the root of (199/53.4%)
2.	the action of inserting into soil (often referring to settle down in a certain place)	扎根(take root)(17/3.6%)	take root (94/25.2%)
3.	the bottom of a specific object	X-根(X-root)(10/2.1%)	
4.	total eradication	根除(root out)(11/2.3%)	root out (27/7.2%)
5.	the underpinnings of an abstract entity	根基(foundation)(277/59.1%)	
6.	support (often referring to one's position/standing in an election)		root for (56/15%)
Total		468	372

Table 3-1 shows that the number of "Root" metaphors based on ROOT + FOUNDATION = ESSENCE is the largest in Chinese, while the "Root" metaphor of the largest proportion is ROOT = CAUSE in English. The results confirmed that Chinese plant conceptualization is more of a hierarchical structure between parts of the plant, of which root is the baseline. The fact that "Root" metaphors based on ROOT = CAUSE is of the largest proportion in English also proves that English conceptualization of plants is more time-oriented, and the event framework of plant growth is the most frequently focalized feature in the "Plant" metaphor formation. The idea is also supported by the verb-based metaphorical expressions "take root" and "root for". Meanwhile, the "Root" metaphor that ranks the second place in Chinese is ROOT + ORIGIN = CAUSE. The metaphor is 根源 (root cause) in Chinese, "根 = root, 源 = the origin of river", similar to the formation of 根基, in which "根 = root, 基 = foundation". 根源 is also an example of using another image with features related to certain features of the plant to extract and enhance these characteristics of the plant, thus realizing the metaphorical projection from concrete "root" to abstract concepts like "importance" and "cause". In other words, as for the Chinese "Root" metaphors, the attention gapping of root-related features is accomplished by adding more required features from another concrete image, and then the similar features between the two concrete images can be extracted and projected onto a more abstract concept. The cognitive process emulates block-building. When the accumulated required features reached a certain point, the abstract concept can be perceived.

According to the corpus analysis in Chapter 3, we learned that the high-frequent 根 metaphor in Chinese is predominantly represented by 根基 (59.1%). In English, the most frequent metaphorical usage of "root" is to represent "cause", often associated with negative events, in the form of "the root of ..." (53.4%). Citing Austin's classification of conceptual structures, "the root of ..." belongs to a core-type conceptual structure, while 根基 is a typical analogical conceptual structure. Even without considering the meaning construction of the expressions 根基 and "the root of ...", based solely on the formal features of the structures, the core-type structure exhibits a scattering pattern from the center to the periphery, while analogy demonstrates a spatially symmetrical structure. The scattering pattern is characterized by high extension and fuzzy boundaries, while the symmetrical pattern has low extension and clear boundaries. The former is more consistent with linear thinking dominated by time, while the latter possesses attributes of spatially dominated symmetrical thinking.

Next, let us compare the meaning construction of 根基 and "the root of …". 根基 belongs to compound nouns (NN), and its meaning construction occurs through bidirectional cross-domain projection based on metaphorical prominence in the domains of 根 and 基 (Bacerlona, 2000). The relationship between the two conceptual domains, 根 and 基, exhibits a symmetrical correspondence. In English, the interpretation of compound nouns (NN) emphasizes asymmetry. Langacker (1991) proposed the premise of asymmetry between the A-structure and D-structure in lexical valency relationships. However, this symmetrical correspondence exhibited in the Chinese compound noun 根基 cannot be effectively explained. For example, we can ask "What ball?" and receive the answer "soccer ball" or ask "What juice?" and receive the answer "carrot juice", but we cannot ask "What base?" and answer with 根基 (Chen, 2016).

From the meaning construction schema of 根基 (Figure 3-1), it can be observed that the highlighted area in the process of abstracting the meaning of 根基 is the region of clear boundary with the background (indicated by bold ellipses). This relatively salient area corresponds to the conceptual representation of 事物 (things) in cognitive grammar, which suggests that its conceptualization relies more on spatial cognitive domains. Furthermore, the symmetric correspondence between 根 and 基 (represented by dashed lines) is based on the similarity of the spatial distribution between the partial wholes in their respective configurations. This similarity provides a prerequisite for the bidirectional cross-domain mapping, resulting in the meaning of 根基 as a natural outcome of the bidirectional cross-domain mapping.

Chapter 3 Spatial-Temporal Cognition Analysis of Disease Metaphors in English and Chinese

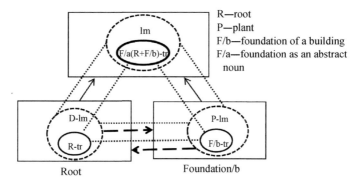

Figure 3-1 Image schema of 根基 in Chinese

The fact that this symmetrical correspondence and construction can be achieved in Chinese precisely illustrates that Chinese relies more on a "synoptic static perspective" to conceptualize a singular configuration of the external world. The imaginary representations of 根 and 基 are positioned based on their respective overall relational patterns, that is, 根 is determined by 植物 (plant) and 基 is determined by 建筑 (building). All the elements contained in 植物 and 建筑 coexist and are simultaneously cognized in the imaginary representations. The spatial distribution characteristics of 根 and 基 within their respective overall imaginary conceptual domains are highlighted. This highlighting allows for the abstraction and extension of meaning in the expressions through four analogical mappings that possess spatial distribution similarity. This can be expressed in formulaic form as:

根(root):植物(plant)＝地基(foundation):建筑(building)
根基(root foundation)＝抽象实体的支撑部分(support for abstract entities)

Analogy is an important means of strengthening linguistic regularity (Saussure, 1959). Juxtaposition itself is a grammatical technique or form. 援物取象 (Xu, 1999) and 对举而言 play important roles in the construction of Chinese NN compound words. By juxtaposing 根 and 基, the semantic filling mechanism is triggered to establish connections. The process of meaning construction involves analogizing the spatial distribution characteristics of different entities within their imaginary overall concepts to generate abstract meanings. Similar 根 metaphors in Chinese include 根源 and 根本 (fundamental), where the surface meanings have detached from the specific meanings of the constituent parts and only express abstract meanings. Such lexical constructions and abstract meanings are common in Chinese, and the analysis of the meaning construction of the NN compound word 根基 in the previous text demonstrates the predominance of a "global static perspective" and spatial cognition in Chinese.

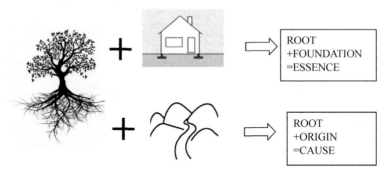

Figure 3-2　Formation process of double-imaged "Root" metaphor in Chinese

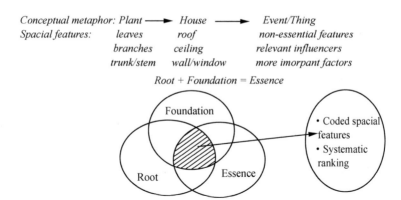

Figure 3-3　Multiple metonymy embedded in the double-imaged metaphorical projection (根基)

Specifically, the meaning "root = cause/origin" is not enhanced and focalized through the paralleled analogy between the concept of a "plant" and a "river", the vertical hierarchical cognition of a plant is complemented with the horizontal development of a river. In this way, the more time-oriented meaning "root = cause" is underscored. Figure 3-1 shows the formation of the Chinese "Root" metaphors: 根基 is usually used to emphasize the importance of things, while 根源 is applied to refer to the cause of some events. It can be seen from Figure 1 the connotative meaning of 根 in Chinese has a more or less balanced distribution between "importance" and "cause", since "root" is both the most essential part of a plant and the very beginning of a plant. The focalization on either of these two relies on the feature accumulation by juxtaposing another image with "root", thus enhancing certain features of root to achieve the cognitive metaphorical projection between "root" and "essence" or "root" and "cause". The metaphorical projection is realized through the accumulation of metonymies construed between different concepts through proximities in certain spatial features and ranking within each correspondent conceptual system. In other words, the metaphor is realized by building metonymic blocks to shorten the distance between the concrete "root" and abstract concepts such as "essence" or "cause" (Shu, 2011). The double-imaged metaphor is also a common way of word formation in Chinese. The accumulation of "metonymic blocks" is itself another evidence for the hypothesis that Chinese is generally more space-oriented in cognition.

Without the integrated image, simply 根 can be used to refer to both reason and essence. Examples can be found in the online Modern Chinese Corpus:

f. 他问我会骑马不会?我没说我会,也没说我不会:他呢,反正找不到别人,也就没究根儿。(老舍,2016:432)

He asked me if I could ride a horse. I didn't say I would, and I didn't say I wouldn't; as for him, he couldn't find anyone else anyway, so he didn't get to the bottom of the matter.

g. "将来,无论走到哪里,家乡都是他的根,系着思念与牵挂。"张平原说。(王永战、吴月,2002)

"In the future, no matter where he goes, his hometown will always be his root, intertwined with his yearn and concern." Zhang Pingyuan said.

In Sentence f, "root" is the metaphorical expression for reasons, while in Sentence g, "root" should be understood as "the essence" of the man according to the context. It is evident that without being combined with other images, the connotative meaning of "root" is flexible and largely depends on the context. However, according to the statistics of Table 3-1, a larger number (59.1%) of the "Root" metaphors are double-imaged metaphors when the "Root" metaphors are enhanced with features from the constructional concept—"foundation", which is in line with the hypothesis that Chinese conceptualization of the "Plant" metaphor is more space-oriented. Yet we have to admit that although less frequently, a plant can also be perceived from a temporal perspective in Chinese such as the 根源 (32.6%), the way of forming this metaphor, as illustrated in Figure 3-1, is the same "metonymic block-building" process adopted in generating a spatial "Plant" metaphor, as shown in Figure 3-2. The formation of double-imaged metaphors relies on the proximity in the spatial features and the similar ranking of these images in their conceptual system. Therefore, only concepts that share a similar hierarchical spacial structure can be easily integrated and used as one metaphorical reference to another more abstract image. The fact that the double-imaged metaphor occupies the majority of "Root" metaphors not only provides evidence of the space-oriented conceptualization of plants in Chinese, but also implies a possible space-oriented cognition of other concepts in general.

Through the analysis of root-oriented disease metaphor translations drawn from the two English translations of *A Dream of Red Mansions*, it is proved that the translation strategies adopted by the two translators are closely associated with the different focus in disease conceptualization between English and Chinese. More cognitive efforts are made in understanding, categorizing, and building a hierarchical structure composed of the spatial features of various components of disease in Chinese, whereas relatively less attention is paid to the involvement of the spatial features of disease as a whole from a temporal perspective. The argument is proved by the translation choices made by Hawks and Yang. The fact that some root-based disease metaphors are not reserved in Hawks' translation yet maintained in Yang's translation can be reasonably explained by the gap between the cognitive efforts distributed to space-oriented characteristics between English and Chinese. When the gap is small, it's very likely that the metaphor can be reserved in the English translation, such as "the root of disease" metaphor. However, when the gap is large, there is a good chance that the metaphorical form would be deserted in the translation, for example, "the root of the family" and "the root of life". The cognitive reasons behind the translation strategies support the argument that Chinese is more space-oriented in plant conceptualization and English is more time-oriented.

The argument has been further proved with statistical analysis of the corpus search results. The "Root" metaphor that accounts for the largest proportion in Chinese is the "root + foundation = importance" metaphor, which emphasizes the spatial features of a plant, and the hierarchical correlation between the components of a plant. On the contrary, the most frequent "Root" metaphor in English is "root = cause", which emphasizes the changes in spatial features from a temporal perspective. Besides, the formation process of relevant "Root" metaphors in Chinese is a feature accumulation process through combing two concepts, which relies more on the space-oriented quantitative cognition. Whether the space-time cognition contrast also exists in the conceptualization of other objects and the reason for the contrast still needs further investigation.

3.3 Spatial-Temporal Cognition of the Word Meaning Construal Between 根 and "Root"

In this section, we hypothesize that the distinction in word meaning extension between Chinese character 根 and its English equivalent "root" is due to the different roles played by space and time in their meaning construal. The study compares the different profilings in the image schema of the metaphorical meaning construction of 根 and "root", proving that the space is the dominant domain in the meaning extension of 根, while time dominates the meaning extension of "root". Besides, by contrasting the perspectival mode in the shematization of 根 and "root", the research reveals that meaning processing of Chinese 根 adopts a static synoptic view, taking the configurational knowledge of the plant as the cognitive boundary, and the temporal cognitive scanning is embedded in the spatial characteristics. Meanwhile, the meaning processing of English "root" adopts a dynamic sequential view, prioritizing the extension of cognitive scanning of "root", and the spacial characteristics of "root" are merely the outcome after the multiplexing and unification of cognitive scanning trail. The different function of space and time in the meaning processing and schematization of 根 and "root" not only provides a deep and general cognitive interpretation for their word meaning differences, but also introduces new perspective in exploring the spacial-temporal view between English and Chinese.

Semantics is the crystallization of experiential conceptualization, while meaning is the process of conceptualization, interpreting objective reality through conventional and customary imagery (Langacker, 1987; Dai, 1990; Chen, 2006; Liu & Wang, 2021). Time and space, as fundamental cognitive abilities of humans (Wang, 2013) and basic cognitive domains (Langacker, 1987), in comparison to the temporal and spatial traces that exist in linguistic forms, have a greater presence in the process of conceptualization, specifically in dynamic meaning construction. Therefore, starting from the process of meaning construction extended from lexical semantics, we can more accurately grasp the role of time and space in cognitive processing within the immediate scope of their influence.

The evolution of lexical semantics is also the result of applying spatio-temporal perceptual abilities to experiential conceptualization. According to the theory of cognitive systems and their interplay (Talmy, 2000), the linguistic system and other human perceptual systems exhibit a corresponding relationship with classificatory spatial structure. Thus, by analyzing the magnitude of the role of time and space in lexical meaning construction, we can to some extent reflect the differences in the status of time and space in cognitive processing among members of a language community. Different languages reflect different ways of thinking and worldview (Lakoff & Johnson, 1980; Langacker, 1987; Humboldt, 1999). Furthermore, the characteristics of a language can only be revealed through comparison with other languages, and it is only through comparing different languages that the commonalities hidden behind their specific traits can be uncovered (Xu, 1999). Therefore, by comparing the process of meaning construction in the semantic extension of English and Chinese vocabulary, we may better understand the differences in the status of time and space in general cognition between English and Chinese, which can definitely shed light on understanding of disease conceptualization between English and Chinese.

Metaphor, as an important mechanism in the semantic extension of vocabulary, is particularly noteworthy because it guides the process of ascent from experience to language (Chen, 2003). "Dead" metaphors in particular, due to the intertwining and transformation of literal and implied meanings, serve as "living fossils" in the study of meaning construction processes. Metaphor is characterized by selective highlighting and image association (Lakoff & Johnson, 1980), and

Chapter 3 Spatial-Temporal Cognition Analysis of Disease Metaphors in English and Chinese

the choice of which part to highlight and how to establish associations between images depends on the conventional usage within a language community, or common sense, as well as Talmy's (2000) emphasized patterned pre-selection. The differences in conventional usage, common sense, and patterned pre-selection among different languages reflect the distinct cognitive processing styles of different ethnic groups, and the differences in the magnitude of the role of time and space in meaning construction are important factors influencing cognitive processing. This study takes the basic equivalent words "root" in English and 根 in Chinese as examples, and comparatively analyzes the meaning construction relying on metaphor in the semantic extension of "root" and 根. By comparing the different types of cognitive processing involved in meaning construction using Langacker's image-schematic model and Talmy's schematic system theory, this study aims to reveal the differences in the status of time and space in the conceptualization of the same object between English and Chinese. Through in-depth exploration of the reasons behind the differences in cognitive processing styles, the following conclusions are drawn: Chinese exhibits a homomorphism between time and space, with time residing in space; whereas in English, time precedes space, and time and space are unified within time.

  The essence of the comparative study of cognitive differences between English and Chinese in the spatio-temporal domain lies in revealing differences in cognitive patterns through the comparison of language. This research topic belongs to the scope of studying the relationship between language, thought, and reality, which is a philosophical proposition. It is also an important topic in the field of contrastive linguistics.

  The comparative study of spatiotemporal cognition between English and Chinese can be broadly divided into two directions: form and meaning. In the late 1980s, with the rise of cognitive linguistics, research based on cognitive foundations began to focus on the unique characteristics of Chinese as a semantically oriented language. It explored the shared aspects of human perception of space and time through language. Researchers investigated the grammatical structure of the Chinese temporal system (Chen, 1988), established the framework of functional grammar for Chinese (Dai, 1990), and explored the cognitive basis of spatial-temporal reference in Chinese (Xu, 1999).

However, in the following decade, the comparative study of spatiotemporal cognition between English and Chinese, based on the unique characteristics of Chinese, did not receive sufficient attention. It was not until Wang (2013) reintroduced this topic into people's attention that the exploration of spatiotemporal cognition in English and Chinese shifted towards a focus on formal comparison rather than semantic analysis. Specifically, the research focused on four aspects: Chinese characters, vocabulary, syntax, and discourse. Through comparing the written features of Chinese characters that combine form and meaning with the phonetic coding system of English (Wang, 2013; He & Wang, 2016a), the diachronic evolution of English and Chinese word formation (Wang & Yu, 2016), English and Chinese word order, syntactic structures, and tense features (Wang, 2013; Ruan & Wang, 2015; Wang & Wang, 2018), as well as the discreteness of Chinese discourse structure and the continuity of English discourse (Wang & He, 2016, 2017), researchers aimed to demonstrate the spatial characteristics of Chinese and the temporal characteristics of English.

According to Xu's (1999) hierarchical classification of non-linear linguistic structures, the series of studies by Wang and his collaborators can be categorized into the levels of formal grammar, representational level, and semantic relationship level of basic structural units. However, these studies lack sufficient attention to the deep level of conceptual semantics in the comparative analysis of English and Chinese.

The English words and Chinese characters can be considered as fundamental structural units in their respective languages, combining form and meaning (Xu, 1999). When comparing the spatio-temporal cognition of English and Chinese in terms of words and characters, it is crucial to pay attention to the level of conceptual semantics rather than being confined to the analysis of formal aspects. Existing studies on lexical comparison tend to prioritize form over meaning, emphasizing morphological differences rather than semantic analysis. These studies often adopt the framework of word-category grammar from Indo-European language theory, assuming that nouns are associated with space and verbs with time. They explore the diachronic evolution of English and Chinese word formation, syntactic features, noun-verb relationships, status, and noun-verb transformations (Wang, 2013; He & Wang, 2016a, 2016b) to conclude that English emphasizes time while Chinese emphasizes space. Some scholars proposed the "noun-verb containment" theory in Chinese word-class issues and considered the differences in English and Chinese thinking patterns from the perspective of noun-verb relationships, suggesting that Chinese "things" contain "events", while English emphasizes the separation of "events" and "things."

The author of this book agrees with the basic viewpoints on the temporal nature of English, the spatial nature of Chinese, and the theory that verb contains noun. However, it argues that the existing research has a tendency to prioritize form over meaning and results over processes in its perspective. Particularly, lexical studies are limited to the comparison of nouns and verbs, oversimplifying complex issues and adopting a correspondence or reflection view of language and reality. However, language and reality do not have a one-to-one correspondence; reality is conceptualized at the level of language, or we can say that language is the encoding of reality (Xu, 1999). Since language is encoding, and conclusions cannot solely be drawn from differences in encoding but should focus on the process of encoding. Although nouns and verbs are applicable to describing reality, they do not correspond directly to the objective reality. Studying spatiotemporal cognition by taking nouns and verbs as the central categories cannot avoid the pitfalls of simple correspondence in the semantic reference theory. Furthermore, while English has clear categorization of nouns and verbs, the categorization of word classes in Chinese has been a topic of ongoing debate (Dai, 1990; Xu, 1999). Thus, using the categorization of nouns and verbs as the basis for English-Chinese comparison subjects to disputes since it lacks the commonality required for comparison. Moreover, the comparison of spatio-temporal cognition between English and Chinese on an unstable foundation inevitably weakens the credibility of the conclusions. The cognitive traces of spatio-temporal cognition indeed leave imprints in static language forms and symbols, but they play a more significant role in dynamic participation in meaning construction. That is, they exert various impacts on the conceptualization of the world and the cognitive processing of the objective world through schema-based cognition. The existing studies mostly tend to treat language as a mirror of reality and overlook the analysis of meaning construction or cognitive processing. It is necessary to incorporate a semantic perspective and compare the differences in the role of time and space in meaning construction or cognitive processing between English and Chinese to gain a clearer and deeper understanding of why English emphasizes time while Chinese emphasizes space, as well as the relationship between time and space in the conceptualization of disease in both languages.

In recent years, there have been two new trends in the research on the comparative analysis of spatial and temporal cognition between English and Chinese. There is a closer integration with the second language acquisition, which explains the underlying cognitive reasons behind common errors or difficulties of Chinese English learners in acquiring English syntactic structures, tense and aspect, and anaphoric expressions from the perspectives of spatial characteristics in Chinese and temporal characteristics in English (Zhao & Wang, 2017; Yang & Wang, 2017). Such research also provides empirical evidence for the conclusions drawn regarding the spatial-temporal differences between English and Chinese in the process of language acquisition.

The comparison between root-based disease metaphors in English and Chinese furthers our understanding of the role of basic domains like space and time played in the conceptualization of disease. An exploration of spatio-temporal cognition between English and Chinese can provide more fundamental cognitive reasons for the different perspectives adopted in treating the common disease between the two cultures.

Chapter 4

Similarities and Differences in the Schematization of Disease and 疾

There is an increasing emphasis on the semantic perspective in exploring the cognitive differences between English and Chinese in terms of lexical spatial and temporal cognition. This includes Wang & Zhang's (2019) analysis of the semantic evolution and lexicalization process of the Chinese negation representation "meiyou" (没有) and their exploration of the cognitive rationale behind the collocation differences between English and Chinese in negation representation. Other studies, such as Cui & Wang's (2019) explanation of the temporal and cognitive differences in the expression of certain verbs between Chinese and English, and Liu & Wang's (2021) comparison between the semantic expressions of English conceptual behavior and Chinese objectification, also paid more attention to the comparison of lexical semantics in the discussion of English-Chinese spatiotemporal issues. Additionally, Liu & Xu (2019) have proposed the concept of Chinese spatiotemporal isomorphism based on the analysis of conflicts in Chinese temporal conceptualization, providing linguistic facts and cognitive evidence for the hypothesis of Chinese spatiotemporal isomorphism and the assumption of English spatiotemporal disjunction, considering the cultural origins, written structures, and grammar systems of English and Chinese. Related research also includes discussions on the boundaries of semantic meanings of Chinese quantifiers (Liu & Li, 2020) and a comparison of the different semantic restrictions on noun-verb sentence conditions between English and Chinese (Ou & Liu, 2021). In contrast to mere formal comparisons and descriptions, analyzing the role of spatiotemporal concepts in cognitive processing from a semantic perspective provides more explanatory power.

This section follows the second new trend in recent years, which is to explain the spatiotemporal cognitive differences through the comparison of lexical semantics in English and Chinese. The previous research from the same perspective has provided inspiration and ideas for this book, but further in-depth advancement is still needed. Firstly, although the assertion by Wang et al. about the spatial thinking in Chinese and the temporal thinking in English provides an overall summary of the different emphases on time and space in English and Chinese, it does not clarify the relationship between time and space. The notion of Chinese spatiotemporal isomorphism proposed by Liu et al. based on the theory of "noun includes verb" is a strong supplement to the subjective viewpoint of Chinese spatial thinking, and the two are not conflicting but can rather be combined as Chinese spatiotemporal isomorphism with an accent on space. However, the view of English spatiotemporal disjunction by Liu et al. is a simple generalization of English characteristics under the framework of Chinese spatial thinking. The concept of "spatiotemporal disjunction" easily leads to the misunderstanding that "time" and "space" are completely separated in English thinking, whereas in reality, English thinking prioritizes time and exhibits a sequential characteristic in cognitive processing, with time and space not being disjointed but unified within the flow of time.

The meaning of words is derived from their cognitive concepts, and different semantic meanings correspond to different cognitive concepts. Therefore, studying the semantic restrictions of words can help us better understand the cognitive differences between English and Chinese in spatial and temporal domains. In Chinese, the noun-verb sentence imposes restrictions on the semantic meanings of words, so it is worth exploring whether English, which lacks such constraints, has more diverse semantic meanings in the spatial and temporal domains. Additionally, the quantitative meaning of Chinese quantifiers also exhibits a rich spatial feature, which calls for further investigation to determine whether English quantifiers have similar characteristics. Furthermore, studying the semantic restrictions of Chinese negation expressions and verb expressions can provide insights into the cognitive differences between English and Chinese in the temporal domain.

To summarize, recent research on the comparative analysis of spatial and temporal cognition between English and Chinese has witnessed two new trends: a

Chapter 4 Similarities and Differences in the Schematization of Disease and 疾

closer integration with the second language acquisition and an increasing emphasis on the semantic perspective. The integration with the second language acquisition explains the cognitive reasons behind common errors or difficulties encountered by Chinese English learners, while the semantic perspective explores the cognitive differences between English and Chinese in terms of the spatial and temporal cognition at the lexical level. These research directions shed light on the underlying cognitive mechanisms and provide valuable insights for understanding the spatiotemporal differences between English and Chinese. However, further research is needed to deepen our understanding of the relationship between time and space, the semantic restrictions of words, and the cognitive differences in the temporal domain.

4.1 Space-Oriented Cognition in Chinese vs Time-Oriented Cognition in English

Saussure (1959) pointed out that language is a collective product of a linguistic community, and Humboldt (1999) emphasized that a kind of language reflects a unique thinking paradigm through which a nation perceives and understands the world, highlighting the close connection among language, culture and cognition. The previous research has demonstrated significant differences in the selection of perceptual reference frames among speakers from different linguistic and cultural backgrounds (Levinson, 1983; Pederson, 1993). This provides a reasonable research foundation for further exploring cognitive differences through language contrast. Cognitive linguistics advocates starting from semantics and exploring the cognitive universals and cultural variations inherent in language along a new path (Liu & Wang, 2021). To study spatiotemporal cognition through semantics, it is necessary to first differentiate among concepts, meanings, and semantics. Concepts are the abstractions of subjective perception and experience, meanings are the conceptualization processes, and semantics refers to a conceptual structure that is habitually used and socially agreed upon. Semantics, being the relatively stable and concrete aspect among the three, exhibits different cognitive processing characteristics of physical entities in the external world under the influence of pre-selected linguistic and cultural patterns. Through repeated conceptual processing and subsequent refinement, conventionalized semantics is formed (Talmy, 2000). Thus, lexical semantics can serve as an entry point to investigate cognitive processing similarities and differences in the construction of lexical meanings across different languages. The extension of semantic use is based on convention, which can be derived from natural conditions or guided by other conventions. The logical meanings of 根 in Chinese and "root" in English, which refer to the underground part of a plant, are arbitrary. However, the conventions in the process from the basic meaning of 根 to metaphorical expressions like 根基 and 病根 in Chinese, and from the basic meaning of "root" to expressions like "the root of the disease" and "take root" in English, exhibit certain patterns and principles. Conventional usage is the result of specific patterned processing. By comparing the conventions in the metaphorical meanings construction of 根 and "root" in English and Chinese, it is possible to reflect the different cognitive processing modes between the two languages. Moreover, it is widely acknowledged that time and space play fundamental, universal, and crucial roles in cognitive processing (Dai, 1990; Wang, 2013). Therefore, exploring the reasons for the processing mode differences in the construction of metaphorical meanings of 根 and "root" can reveal the different roles played by time and space.

Although cognitive processing is activated by external objective stimuli, the object of cognitive processing is not the external object itself. As Kant stated, the object of cognition is not the thing itself but the phenomenon (Kant, 1908). Similarly, language can only talk about possibilities rather than the actual things, and we understand reality through possibilities. In line with the philosophical understanding of the relationship between language and reality, Talmy (2000) proposed a universal fictive mode of language, and Langacker also used "mental image" to refer to the object of cognitive processing, employing "image schema" to simulate cognitive processing. In the cognitive processing of mental images, Langacker pointed out that the temporal domain and the spatial domain are fundamental cognitive domains in the cognitive matrix, and Talmy emphasized that the domain composed of time and space permeates various other types of schemas. Langacker (1987) further stated that humans typically activate multiple cognitive domains during cognitive processing, with the dominant domain located near the

Chapter 4 Similarities and Differences in the Schematization of Disease and 疾

center, and domains with lower activation levels positioned closer to the periphery, resembling a radial dashboard of domains. Based on this theory, we can concretize the spatiotemporal cognition contrast between English and Chinese as a comparison of the centrality of the temporal domain and the spatial domain within the cognitive domain matrix. This study further narrows down the research focus to the centrality of the temporal domain and the spatial domain in the construction of metaphorical meanings of 根 in Chinese and "root" in English. The comparison of cognitive processing between English and Chinese involves multiple concepts, and the centrality of the temporal and spatial domains is influenced by the selection of attention focus, perspective, and level of abstraction, corresponding to the concepts of viewpoint, viewpoint schemas, and attentional distribution proposed by Talmy (2000).

In this chapter, we first analyzes the metaphorical meaning construction of 根 and "root" based on Langacker's theory of image schemas. The focus is on the differences and similarities in the construction process of the "cognitive profiling". Specifically, we look into which symbolic structure, "thing" or "relations", tends to be highlighted in the image schemas of the 根 and "Root" metaphors. Based on this analysis, in combination with Talmy's configurational structure schema system involving discreteness and boundary concepts, we tend to examine the correspondence between "thing" and "space", as well as "relations" and "time". Given that space and time underlie our cognition of all kinds of things and phenomena a in the world. A further analysis into the spacial-temporal cognition between English and Chinese can help us deepen our understanding of disease cognition between Chinese and English.

In cognitive grammar, the image schema of "thing" is a relatively foregrounded region. This means that the formation of the image schema of "thing" depends on the concept of "boundary", where entities must be a bounded quantity or have the potential to become a bounded quantity. Dai (1990) has pointed out that the concept of forming boundaries primarily relies on spatial-dominant static thinking. Furthermore, according to Talmy's (2000) explication of boundaries and discreteness, the parts within the bounded quantity exhibit stronger continuity and lower discreteness. Therefore, "low discreteness" is also an important factor in the formation of the image schema of "thing" (Langacker,

133

1987). Combining the concepts of boundaries and discreteness, "thing" can be understood as a coexistence of low-discrete unitary entities within a background of high discreteness. When all elements co-occur in a certain relational pattern and are cognitively perceived simultaneously, it precisely aligns with Talmy's (2000) definition of a static state. Thus, the symbolic structure of "thing" in Langacker's image schema can be seen as the result of spatial-dominant static cognition (Figure 4-1).

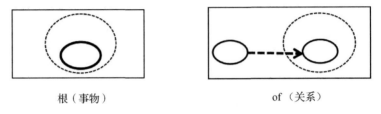

根（事物）　　　　　　　　　　　of（关系）

Figure 4-1 Image schemas of entities and relations (using 根 and "of" as examples)

Time is often considered a more abstract concept than space. Clark (1973) pointed out that if time is metaphorically conceptualized using space, its characteristics can be described as unidirectional, asymmetric, and necessitated by dynamic events. The essence of language lies in distinguishing and connecting, where spatial-dominant cognition primarily serves to "distinguish" entities from the background, while time-dominant cognition primarily serves to "connect" different entities. Therefore, time inherently possesses "directionality". Philosopher Sartre (2001) also interpreted time as an extension of attention in a specific direction. Langacker's image schema of "relations" is represented by an arrow that connects different regions. The arrow schema includes directionality, and its implicitly touchable fictive representation involves fictive motion from one point to another. That is, the points constituting the line appear sequentially rather than simultaneously. Based on the above, the schema of "relations" can be seen as the result of time-dominant dynamic cognition. By establishing the correspondence between "thing" and "space", "relations" and "time", the following section will compare the degree of salience given to "thing" and "relations" in the expression of the 根/root metaphorical image schemas, in order to further understand the centrality of time and space domains in the cognitive processing of disease between English and Chinese.

In different languages, physical entities in the real world may undergo

Chapter 4　Similarities and Differences in the Schematization of Disease and 疾

different schematic processes, and an important factor influencing these processes is the pre-selection of different schemas (Talmy, 2000). In other words, specific languages require a conventionalized way of perceiving certain situations or objects, where certain physical details or characteristics of the objects are idealized and abstracted. The discussion on schematic pre-selection is based on Talmy's proposition of linguistic universal fictiveness, which suggests that in the cognitive representation of a single object, factual representation and fictive representation often exhibit inconsistent characteristics. Moreover, different languages vary in the fictive representation of the same object, and these differences in fictive representation serve as an important entry point for studying cognitive differences among different language groups. Taking "root" in plants as an example, the metaphorical expressions derived from "root", such as 病根 in Chinese and "the root of the disease" in English, have equivalent meanings on the surface. However, the Chinese compound word 病根 is simpler in form, and the reason for the different forms is related to the differences in fictive representation. The surface semantic equivalence between 病根 and "the root of the disease" can be understood as corresponding to the higher palpability level of the factual representation, while differences exist at the lower palpability level of the fictive representation. The differences in cognitive processing at the fictive representation level are primarily manifested in perspective patterns, including perspective point, perspective distance, and the observed direction in the distribution of attention (the perspective point and the observed direction correspond to Langacker's concepts of cognitive location and scanning). Additionally, perspective patterns can be further analyzed in terms of scale (plexity), state of boundedness, and the previously mentioned discreteness.

　　Specifically, perspective patterns can be divided into two types: global static and local dynamic. The global perspective implies that the perspective point is far from the observed object, while the local perspective is the opposite. Based on human perceptual experience, visual perception of distant objects tends to be static, while the observations of close objects are more likely to manifest as dynamic cognition. The global static perspective involves the simultaneous recognition of the entire relational pattern of the observed object, idealizing the observed object as a region composed of internally low discreteness elements, exhibiting characteristics of space-dominant cognition. On the other hand, the local dynamic perspective is the opposite, where the attention window is focused on the line connecting regions rather than the regions themselves. Even for static objects in reality, a local dynamic perspective can be adopted and the process includes the following steps: at first, envision the process of the object's formation, then establish the status of unit entities for each movement through unit extraction, and finally form a model with high internal discreteness through multiplexing and holistic formatting. The local dynamic perspective demonstrates features of directionality and sequentiality, representing a time-dominant processing mode.

After establishing the correspondence between "global static perspective" and "spatial cognition", "local dynamic perspective" and "temporal cognition", the following section uses root-based disease metaphor to argue that the schematic representation of 根 in Chinese abstracts the downward extension characteristic of "roots" and adopts a more space-dependent global static perspective, highlighting the relational pattern between the root and other components of the plant. In contrast, English "root" abstracts the relationship with the trunk as a whole and perceives "root" from a local dynamic perspective, emphasizing the dynamic attribute of the root's underground extension, which is a time-dominant structural historical perception schema.

4.2 Comparison of the Image Schemas of Frequent Disease Metaphors with 根/Root

When we learn a new usage of a word, we focus on language, while when we use a familiar word, we focus on the world. In this sense, the more conventional a word is, the closer it is to our default understanding of the world. This view is consistent with the encyclopedic view of meaning in cognitive linguistics, which suggests that the conventionality of meaning arises from frequent usage, and the centrality of a particular aspect of an object is positively correlated with the degree of fixed expression and its potential for activation. Therefore, high-frequency expressions retrieved from corpora can be considered as highly fixed conventional usages, and the analysis of the meaning construction of these expressions can

Chapter 4 Similarities and Differences in the Schematization of Disease and 疾

reflect the patterned pre-selection and cognitive processing characteristics of the members of the language community. In the following sections, we will take the high-frequency disease metaphors of 根 and "root" as retrieved examples and use the image schema model to conduct a comparative analysis of temporal and spatial cognition between English and Chinese. More specifically, the theoretical framework is based on the conceptual correspondences between "things" and "a static and synoptic view", as well as "relationship" and "a dynamic-partial view".

Contrary to the search results for 根 in the Modern Chinese Corpus, the search results for "root" in the COCA corpus reveal that the high-frequency metaphor is the phrase "the root of …", which is often used to refer to the cause of negative consequences. Although "the root of something" is nominally a noun phrase, with the factual representation of the metaphor being "something", its meaning construction or imaginary representation emphasizes the "connection" between things rather than the things themselves. Let's analyze the example of "the root of disease" while comparing it to the corresponding Chinese metaphorical image schema of 病根 (Figure 4-2 and Figure 4-3).

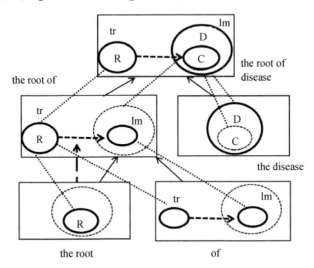

Figure 4-2 The root of disease in English

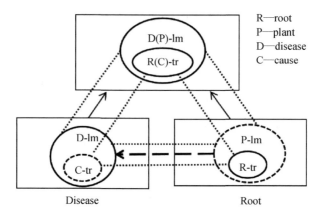

Figure 4-3 病根 in Chinese

Figures 4-2 and 4-3 provide schematic analyses of the construction of meaning for "the root of disease" and 病根 respectively. Through comparison, the most significant difference in the two schemas lies in the symbolic structure that is being emphasized, whether it is "things" or "relationships". In both cases, the representation of "things" is depicted in bold, highlighted circles or ellipses within a specific region, while the "relationships" between "things" are represented by short dotted lines with arrows.

Figure 4-3 illustrates that in the meaning construction of "the root of disease", the emphasis lies in the temporal "relationship" between the trajector-tr (root) and the landmark-lm (disease). The highlighting of "things" aims to reveal the "relationship", that is, the emphasis is on the "line" with the direction between two points rather than the "points" themselves. Additionally, the cross-domain mapping (long dotted line with arrow) externalizes the relationship between "Root (R)" and "Plant (P)" through the schema of "of", resulting in the final schema being a "relationship" schema rather than an emphasis on the attributes of "things". In other words, the construction of meaning in "the root of disease" relies on the dynamic similarity with specific attentional directionality, where "root" grows into "plant" and "cause" leads to "disease". It adopts a "local dynamic perspective" that focuses on the dynamic extension of "root" underground and the process of "cause" inducing disease, while closing the window of attention on "plant" and "disease".

From a logical causality perspective, "the root of disease" emphasizes the

Chapter 4 Similarities and Differences in the Schematization of Disease and 疾

dynamic cause of the "disease", which can be expressed by the following formula:

Root → *Plant* = **Cause** → *Disease*

Root → *Disease* (the root of the disease)

However, in Figure 4-3, the cross-domain mapping for the Chinese expression 病根 is similar to the previous analysis of 根基 in Figure 4-1, as it is based on the spatial configuration similarity between 病因 and 疾病 with 根 and 植物. Although the meaning construction of 病根 and 根基 is not identical, the cross-domain mapping in 病根 is unidirectional rather than bidirectional. However, both conceptual domains still rely on the analogy of spatial distribution features to construct the meaning of 病根.

In the meaning construction process, the procedural "relationship" attribute of the growth from 根 to 植物 in 病根 is relatively backgrounded or abstracted. It emphasizes the attribute of "things", namely the highlighted specific region relative to the background domain (represented by the bold elliptical region). From a logical causality perspective, 病根 emphasizes the causal essence of the "disease" and can be expressed as:

病 (disease): 病因 (cause) = 植物 (plant): 根 (root)

病 (disease): 根 (root)

The comparative analysis of the conceptual schemas of 病根 and "the root of disease" in Chinese and English demonstrates the different focuses on "things" and "relationships". Additionally, Langacker (1987) emphasizes that semantic description should describe not only the constituent elements but also the paths of combination. The emphasis on "relationship" in English can be further explained by Langacker's concept of "valence". Using the examples of "corn kernel" and "kernel of the corn", Langacker illustrated that the use of the preposition "of" in "kernel of the corn" highlights the "relationship" between a particular configuration and the overall structure. Similarly, in the English expression "the root of disease", the usage of "of" highlights the "relationship" attribute. Specifically, "the root of disease" involves two layers of valence relations. In the first layer, the valence between "the root" and "of" determines the non-temporal relationship, with the preposition "of" highlighting this aspect. Although in the second layer, "disease" serves as the determining element, the entire expression "the root of disease" emphasizes the "relationship" more than " * disease root". It should be noted that " * disease root" is not valid in English, while the valence relation in the Chinese expression 病根 is essentially the same as " * disease root". The substructure of 病 corresponds to the highlighted aspect of 根, which determines the attribute of "things" and explains 根 with the substructure of 病因. Although 病 and 植物 belong to different conceptual domains, the projection of the spatial configuration activated by 根 in the domain of plants is projected onto the abstract concept of 疾病, thereby generating the metaphor of 病根. Similar to 根基, the meaning construction of 病根 emphasizes the attribute of "things" rather than "relationships" (Figures 4-2 and 4-3).

By analyzing the high-frequency disease metaphors of "root" and 根, namely 病根, "the root of disease", and the comparative analysis of the meaning construction schemas and valence relations corresponding to the metaphor of 病根, we can now conclude that the meaning construction of 病根 focuses on the attribute of "things" and tends to adopt a static and synoptic perspective to construct the meaning of the constituent parts from an overall spatial configuration. On the other hand, the meaning construction of "the root of disease" emphasizes "relationships" and tends to adopt a partial and dynamic perspective to reconstruct the linear process of root growth. Considering that "things" and "a static and synotic perspective" reflect the dominance of spatial cognition, while "relationships" and "a partial dynamic perspective" reflect the dominance of temporal cognition, we can infer that the semantic extension processing of 根 in Chinese is primarily guided by spatial factors, while the semantic processing of "root" in English relies more on temporal factors.

4.3 Differences in Schematization of the Disease Metaphor with 根 and "Root"

4.3.1 Differences in Perspectival Mode for 根 and "Root"

In the process of schema processing in a language, certain details of a specific physical entity may be abstracted (Talmy, 2000). The symbolic meaning constructed

Chapter 4 Similarities and Differences in the Schematization of Disease and 疾

through schema processing is strengthened with each use, and as the degree of its solidification increases, the corresponding schema processing method also deepens. The corpus retrieval results mentioned earlier show that the Chinese compound word 根基 has a very high frequency of use in Chinese. In the process of constructing its meaning, it relies on a synoptic and static perspective, highlighting the relative spatial positioning features of 根 and 基 in the overall spatial configurations.

However, unlike buildings, the growth of plants in the real world includes both upward growth (Up) and the downward extension of their roots into the ground (Down) (Figure 4-4). In the metaphorical construction of the meaning of 根基, the attention window is focused on the spatial distribution features of 根 and 基 relative to 植物 and 建筑, emphasizing an upward cognitive scan (Up) and relatively backgrounding the downward extension of 根 from the ground (Ground-G) (Down). The viewpoint or cognitive orientation (Orientation-O) for observing 根 also shifts from the ground (G) to the bottom of 根. Due to the high frequency of usage of 根基 in Chinese, the deepening of its solidification also leads to the completion of the conceptualization of 根 from Schema A to Schema B. Compared with Schema A, Schema B blurs the segmentation of the plant by the ground level, and the downward shift in cognitive orientation (O) relies more on the knowledge of the overall configuration of 根 in relation to the plant, highlighting an upward cognitive scan (Up). Overall, compared with Schema A, the cognitive scanning direction of 根 image is more consistent in Schema B. The dispersion between internal elements is reduced. The region has a higher salience relative to the background, and it is easier to activate the spatial domain and form a concept of 事物.

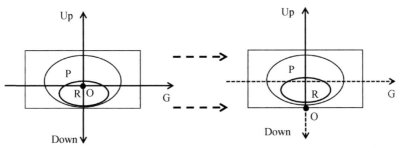

Figure 4-4 Changes in cognitive scanning direction in the schema processing of the Chinese word 根

Cognitive and Contrastive Analysis of Disease Metaphors in English and Chinese

　　As shown in Figure 4-4, 根基 as the most frequently used metaphor in Chinese strengthens the consistency of cognitive scanning direction for the concept of 根 in Chinese, reducing the dispersion within the attention window, and facilitates the prioritized activation of the spatial domain for conceptualization. The result of conceptualizing 根 based on the spatial domain also highlights the "thing" attribute of 根. The downward shift in cognitive orientation (O) and the emphasis on upward cognitive scanning in Chinese reinforce the spatial positioning characteristics of 根 relative to the overall plant. Based on this salient feature, the meaning of the Chinese word 根 is extended and abstracted. Chinese 根 can refer to the connecting area of a three-dimensional physical entity, whose height outweighs its width, to the ground, even including the zone above the connecting area deviating from the prototype meaning of "being underground". For example, Chinese expressions 墙根 (wall root), which refers to the connection between a wall and the ground and the upward part, and 窗根 (window root), which refers to the connection between a window and the wall or ground and the upward part. However, the corresponding English expressions are not widely accepted. Whether translated as "wall root" and "window root", or as "the root of the wall" or "the root of the window", they cannot be universally understood. The reason for this is that the comprehension of expressions like 墙根 and 窗根 requires the abstraction of the meaning construction of 根 to include the abstracted features of "underground" or "invisible" and the establishment of an idealized model that highlights the spatial configuration knowledge of 根 in relation to the whole entity. Otherwise, it is difficult to comprehend. The analysis of the conceptual image schema of "the root of disease" (Figure 4-3) mentioned earlier shows that the cognitive processing of "root" in English highlights the dynamic process of downward extension, and based on Talmy's assessment of the universal fictive models in language, it can be said that the fictive motion associated with the comprehension of "root" in English is the motion of extending downward, backgrounding its connection with the above-ground parts of the plant. Therefore, it cannot activate the meaning construction of "root" referring to visible entities above the ground.

Chapter 4 Similarities and Differences in the Schematization of Disease and 疾

4.3.2 Synoptic Static Perspectival Mode vs Partial Dynamic Perspectival Mode

In the previous discussion, Figures 4-3 and 4-4 compared the conceptual image schemas of "the root of disease" and 病根 respectively. It was found that the meaning construction of "the root of the disease" highlights the "relationship" between entities, while 病根 emphasizes the entity itself. The following comparison of perspective modes and attention distribution in the cognitive processing of 病根 and "the root of disease" aims to enhance the understanding of spatiotemporal concepts in English and Chinese. It specifically involves variables such as cognitive orientation, cognitive scanning, dispersion, and level of conceptual implication.

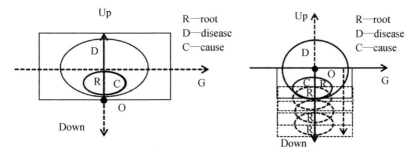

Figure 4-5 Cognitive orientation and scanning of 病根

Figure 4-6 Cognitive orientation and scanning of "the root of disease"

Figure 4-4 in the above text illustrates that in Chinese, the ultimate conceptual image schema expression of 病根 emphasizes the attribute of "thing", specifically the area that is highlighted relative to the background. Given that the determining component of 病根 in the construction of its meaning is 根, the conceptualization involves a cross-domain projection from the spatial configuration knowledge of the plant to the concept of disease. Therefore, in Figure 4-6, the cognitive orientation and scanning of 病根 continue the characteristics of 根 in Figure 4-5, including the downward shift in cognitive orientation (Orientation-O), the emphasis on upward (Up) cognitive scanning direction, and the blurring of the ground division line (G) and downward (Down) cognitive scanning. The attention window covers all elements within the conceptual domain, including the fictional representations of 根 and the partial holistic relationship patterns between 根 and 疾病, as well as the cognitive scanning of upward extension. Moreover, due to the consistency in the extension direction of cognitive scanning and the blurring of the ground division line, the discreteness between the elements within the attention window is reduced, forming a concept with clearer boundaries. The cognitive orientation and scanning features of 病根 indicate that its schematic processing in Chinese adopts a synoptic static perspective primarily based on spatial domain. All elements of the fictional representation of the plant as an entity, including the cognitive scanning of upward extension, are within the attention window, suggesting that the conceptualization of 病根 in Chinese is spatiotemporally homomorphic. At the same time, the range of the attention window is determined by the boundaries evoked by the plant as an entity, and the linear extension of cognitive scanning is limited by this boundary. Therefore, although it is spatiotemporally homomorphic, spatial dominance is predominant.

In contrast, Figure 4-5 in the previous context demonstrates that in English, the metaphor "the root of disease" highlights the characteristic of "root" being below the ground level (G) and continuously extending downward. The cognitive orientation (Orientation-O) of "root" remains on the highlighted ground division line, and the part-whole relationship between "root" and the plant as well as the upward cognitive scanning are relatively backgrounded. The backgrounding or abstraction of the part-whole relationship between "root" and the plant is also reflected in the English expression for "the roots of tree". The English expression of the concept cannot simply be translated as "the root of tree". The corpus retrieval results show that the plural form of "root", i.e. "roots", must be used in English expressions of the concept, namely "the roots of tree". However, the fact that "the root of disease" is not valid indicates that the schematic processing of "the root of disease" is not based on the part-whole relationship between "root" and "tree". Additionally, the analysis of the conceptual image schema in Figure 4-3 also indicates that "the root of disease" emphasizes the "relationship" rather than the "entity" in its meaning construction. The entities within the attention window are involved in a process of extension from point to line, which involves a series of cognitive processes. Each extension of "root" is initially bounded as a unit entity and then undergoes multiplexing, followed by a sequential downward movement of the partial or narrowed attention window, gradually perceiving multiple unit

Chapter 4 Similarities and Differences in the Schematization of Disease and 疾

entities, and ultimately achieving the formation of the entire Gestalt. Although the final processed result of "the root of disease" is a complex of "linear models", the processing adopts a local dynamic perspective, with the directional extension of the attention window playing a dominant role. The ultimate holistic linear model is presented as attention extends downward, with high discreteness among elements within the conceptual domain and an unclear overall boundary. These processing characteristics reflect the dominance of time in English cognition, where time and space are unified within time domain.

In the process of schematic processing, the metaphorical representation evoked by "the root of disease" emphasizes the dynamic process of downward growth of the plant's "root". The metaphorical representation evoked by 病根 in Chinese focuses on the position of the root within the entire plant based on the pattern of part-whole relationship. Figure 4-5 illustrates that the cognitive scanning direction of the concepts 根 and 病 in the metaphor of 病根 is consistent, indicating a low level of discreteness among the conceptual representations and facilitating the activation of a holistic boundary perception, thereby forming a spatially dominant understanding of "thingness". Conversely, Figure 6 shows that the cognitive scanning direction of the concepts "Root (R)" and "Disease (D)" in the metaphor "the root of disease" is opposite, indicating a higher level of discreteness among the conceptual representations, making it difficult to activate a holistic boundary, and emphasizing the individuated state of each representation. These findings further support the conclusion drawn earlier regarding the predominance of a local dynamic framework in English conceptual processing.

The low discreteness within 病根 and the high discreteness within the metaphor of "the root of disease" can also be explained in conjunction with the degree of conceptual implication in language. Similar concepts in different languages are often expressed using different linguistic forms. What is implied in one language may be explicitly expressed in another language. For instance, the construction of the metaphorical meaning of 病根 in Chinese relies on the part-whole relationship between 根 and 病. However, this relationship is implicit and lacks explicit linguistic form. In contrast, the equivalent expression in English, "the root of disease", formalizes the relationship using the preposition "of". The reason for the difference in formalized expression between two similar concepts lies in the entanglement of concepts within the source domain of the metaphor. In the case of 病根, the lack of a clear and distinct boundary for 根 compared to 植物 (as indicated by the virtualization of the ground division line) results in an entanglement of the concepts within the target domain of 疾病. Due to the absence of clear boundaries between concepts, their relationship cannot be formalized. In contrast, the possibility of formalizing the relationship using the preposition "of" in English stems from the distinct boundary between "root" and "plant" with the ground division line being consistently emphasized during the semantic extension of "root". The clear boundaries between the two concepts provide a prerequisite for formalizing their relationship, leading to the expression "the root of disease" in English, while precluding the use of the possessive form that typically signifies a closer possession relationship ("disease's root") or a direct correspondence to the Chinese expression ("disease root").

Things are "spoken out" at different levels of conceptual implication, and the differences in formal expression between 病根 and "the root of disease" reflect the varying degrees of conceptual implication. In the construction of the meaning of 病根, the conceptual "relationships" are backgrounded, and all elements, including the upward cognitive scanning, coexist within the same attentional window, resulting in low discreteness among the elements within the domain and a high degree of conceptual implication. This facilitates the formation of a bounded quantity of cognition and activates a synoptic static perspective dominated by space. Similarly, the fact that "the root of disease" can be described using an independent linguistic form (the preposition "of") implies a lower degree of conceptual implication and higher discreteness among the elements within the domain. The nature of the cognitive scanning direction between "root" and "plant", where the attention window moves sequentially in the direction of root growth, relies on a locally dynamic perspective dominated by time. The complex configuration of the whole organism becomes evident as time progresses. The analysis of cognitive scanning, cognitive localization, internal element discreteness, and degree of conceptual implication in 病根 and "the root of disease" further corroborates the aforementioned conclusions regarding the spatial-temporal cognition in English and Chinese languages.

Chapter 4　Similarities and Differences in the Schematization of Disease and 疾

4.4　Sign Language Evidence for Different Perspectives in Viewing 根 and "Root"

Tamly pointed out that languages can systematically and extensively use their own forms and constructions that represent motion to describe static scenes, which is called constructional fictive motion. He also noted that individuals may differ in the intensity of their perception of this fictive motion. Based on the comparison of the perspective modes and attention distribution of 病根 and "the root of disease" in the previous discussion, it was concluded that English tends to adopt a local dynamic perspective in the schematic processing of "root", emphasizing the conceptualization of the root's growth process and highlighting the underground and downward extension characteristics of the root. On the other hand, Chinese employs a synoptic static perspective in the schematization of 根, relying on overall spatial configuration knowledge of plants to locate the root, emphasizing its role as a connected component at the bottom of the plant. Combining Talmy's discussion on fictive motion, we can reasonably infer that the English phrase "the root of disease" implies a stronger fictive motion originating from the front end of "root", while the perception of this fictive motion from the root in Chinese is relatively weaker. The similarities and differences in the schematic processing of 根/root between English and Chinese can also be found in the expression of 根 and "root" in Sign Language.

The dynamic nature of the expression of "root" in American Sign Language (ASL), as shown in Figure 4-7, reflects the emphasis on the growth process of "root" in English. In ASL, to express "root", the signer first forms the sign for the number "4" with both hands, keeps the non-dominant hand stable with the palm facing upward (symbolizing the ground), and vertically lowers the dominant hand into the non-dominant hand (symbolizing the downward growth process of "root"). The dynamic expression in the Sign Language of "root" highlights the growth process of "root" in English, and the non-dominant hand serving as the ground that divides the plant into above-ground and underground parts, which also emphasizes the underground feature of "root". In contrast, the Sign Language expression of 根 in Chinese is quite different, as shown in Figure 4-8. To express 根 in Chinese Sign Language, one needs to let the right hand hang down with fingers spread open and pointing towards the ground (activating the overall plant configuration), and then hold the right wrist with the left hand and keep it still. In the entire Sign Language expression, the open fingers representing 根 do not move at all, and the gesture of the left hand holding the right wrist does not highlight the division of the plant from the ground but serves as a connecting link within the overall plant configuration, not affecting the overall plant configuration. The meaning construction of 根 in Chinese Sign Language first activates the overall plant configuration knowledge and then achieves the spatial positioning of 根 relative to the overall plant. The different expressions of "root" and 根 in English and Chinese Sign Languages further corroborate the earlier conclusion that the meaning construction of English "root" relies more on the temporal domain, conceptualizing the dynamic growth process of "root", while the meaning construction of Chinese 根 is predominantly driven by the spatial domain, establishing an idealized model of 根 in relation to the overall spatial configuration of the plant.

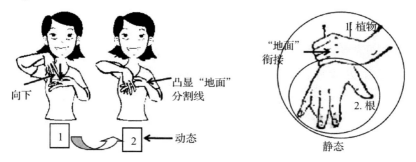

Figure 4-7　ASL for "root"　　　　**Figure 4-8　Chinese Sign Language for 根**

With the intention of further investigating the spatio-temporal features in the conceptualization of disease between English and Chinese, this chapter has explored the cognitive differences in the conceptualization of the same object (plant roots) in English and Chinese, focusing on the meaning construction process. Specifically, starting from the semantic extension of the vocabulary 根/root, which is often used to indicate the cause for the disease, the chapter analyzed and compared the cognitive processing characteristics related to attention distribution

Chapter 4 Similarities and Differences in the Schematization of Disease and 疾

(emphasizing "entities" vs "relationships") and perspective patterns (synoptic-static vs partial-dynamic) that are manifested in the process of schematic processing in English and Chinese.

The analysis reveals that Chinese tends to adopt a synoptic-static perspective, using spatial configuration knowledge of plants to construct an idealized representation of the "thing" attributes of roots, abstracting the process of downward extension and aligning cognitive scanning with the distribution of the boundaries of "thing" in plants. The cognitive processing exhibits spatiotemporal homomorphism, emphasizing the unity of time and space. In contrast, English tends to adopt a partial-dynamic perspective, conceptualizing the downward growth process of "root" through predominantly temporal cognition, highlighting the directional "relationship" property from point to line. The attention window unfolds sequentially as the "root" extends downward, ultimately forming a "linear model" through holistic formalization. This reflects the result of individual motion boundedness and diversification, with the cognitive processing of English centered around time.

Furthermore, the argument regarding the contrasting relationship between the degree of conceptual implication and discreteness further explains, from a theoretical perspective, why the conceptualization of 根 in Chinese relies more on space, while "root" in English focuses on time. The comparison of the characteristics of 根/root in Sign Languages also provides empirical evidence for this conclusion. The deeper analysis of the spatio-temporal cognitive features of "root" and 根 between English and Chinese can shed light on our understanding of disease conceptualization. Based on the comparative analysis, we can deduce that Chinese tends to view disease more as an object or thing, while English is prone to perceive disease as a process.

149

Chapter 5

Social-Cultural Analysis of Differences in Expressing Causes of Diseases in English and Chinese

Linguistic meaning possesses an encyclopedic quality (Langacker, 1987), extending beyond mere lexical definitions. Furthermore, words serve as prompts that elicit intricate conceptualization and act as gateways to comprehensive knowledge. The meanings of metaphorical mappings should not be confined solely to the lexical level; instead, they arise from complex conceptualization constructed through linguistic constructions. Within the context of Covid-19, the use of disease metaphors can streamline cognitive efforts involved in conceptualizing and comprehending novel entities and intricate issues, while also appealing to the emotions and evaluations of the public, thereby eliciting their support and criticism. Notably, the emergence of these deliberate metaphors in cognition and their effectiveness in communication during the pandemic depend on the public's familiarity with the context and their shared experiences derived from the physical environment and socio-cultural situations.

The corpus-based analysis of disease metaphors in English and Chinese reveals that the perception of "disease" varies across cultures. Even when employing the same metaphor, there are distinctions in the emphasized semantic features of the source and target domains. This prompts the following question: Why do these differences exist? Chapter 4 addressed this question from a cognitive perspective by contrasting the spatio-temporal cognitive schema employed in the "Plant" metaphor and examining the process of meaning construction in the Chinese character 根 and its English equivalent "root". Through analyzing the meaning of 根 and "root", a significant divergence in the cognition of disease between English and Chinese becomes evident, specifically in relation to the causes of diseases. Consequently,

Chapter 5 Social-Cultural Analysis of Differences in Expressing Causes of Diseases in English and Chinese

the crucial focus lies in understanding the concept of "cause" rather than "disease". In other words, the conceptualization of causative motions differs between English and Chinese, which profoundly impacts the cognition of disease formation and transmission. Thus, this chapter shifts its attention from disease metaphors alone to the expressions of causative motions in English and Chinese.

As causative motions are present in all languages, the diverse expressions utilized in causative constructions can serve as indicators of sociocultural characteristics. By comparing the syntactic and semantic features of causative motions in English and Chinese, we can uncover the socio-cultural elements that have contributed to the formation of specific causative constructions. The analysis of multi-modal examples enhances our understanding of metaphor's role in sense-making and communication during an extraordinary global crisis. Furthermore, it provides fresh insights into metaphor creativity as a multi-dimensional phenomenon that integrates conceptual, discursive, and cultural factors. In this chapter, the author explores the emergence of metaphors in various cultural, social, political, and institutional contexts. This study reveals that the perception of metaphors differs from context to context, highlighting the significance of cultural experience in target domains as crucial variable in metaphor perception and the framing of social phenomena. We anticipate that further research will uncover the metaphorical, metonymic, and symbolic complexities of Covid-19, recognizing it not only as a natural phenomenon but also as a cultural phenomenon that warrants thorough examination and research to develop socially grounded strategies for better managing and coping with the pandemic.

Metaphors can be categorized in different ways. In the previous chapters, metaphor classification primarily focused on the source domain involved in the projection. Alternatively, metaphors can be classified as deliberate or non-deliberate based on intentions and rhetorical effects. Deliberate metaphors emphasize "the intentional use of a metaphor as a metaphor", building upon Steen's three-dimensional taxonomy for metaphor properties (linguistic, conceptual, and communicative), with particular emphasis on the communicative aspect.

It is important to note that the deliberateness of a metaphor at the linguistic level is assessed through its discourse context and a particular purpose on a particular occasion. In exploring deliberate disease metaphors used in target editorials, we consider the contextual factors that influence deliberate choices of source domains and the various pragmatic effects that can be achieved. Deliberate metaphors serve communicative purposes such as attracting attention, simplifying complex issues, implying evaluations, and conveying stances. Meanwhile, non-deliberate metaphors are often closely associated with subconsciousness. A deeper investigation into the cognition underlying causative actions can enhance our understanding of the cognitive and socio-cultural reasons behind the emergence and adoption of specific disease metaphors.

From the reports on China's pandemic situation published by *China Daily* and BBC News, we have come to understand that the language used to talk about Covid-19 is abundant with metaphors. These metaphors form an extensive collection of figurative patterns, which contribute to the generation of social and political meanings. It is highly likely that these meanings will have a lasting impact on our conceptualization and management of pandemic for many years to come. However, our previous corpus-based analysis has primarily focused on the frequency and distribution of specific metaphors, particularly the similarities and differences in how disease is conceptualized in English and Chinese, as well as the associated ideologies and the emotional responses they elicit. Insufficient attention has been given to the perception of disease causes and the public's attitudes towards potential consequences of disease. Therefore, this chapter will focus on the cognitive, social-cultural analysis of expressions for causations in English and Chinese, with an aim of gaining deeper understanding of the attention distribution in interpreting causative motion, which will eventually shed light on the conceptualization of causes for disease in English and Chinese.

5.1 Differences in Expressions for Causative Motions Between English and Chinese

To compare the conceptualization of causes in English and Chinese, we have chosen the typical three-element causative construction in English and the Chinese Ba construction as the objects of study. The constraints imposed on verb access in the English three-element causative action construction, as presented by Goldberg,

Chapter 5 Social-Cultural Analysis of Differences in Expressing Causes of Diseases in English and Chinese

do not apply to Chinese verb sentences. The meaning of the three-element construction in Chinese Ba sentences can be understood as follows:

(1) The word "Ba" in sentences serves as the main indicator of resistance and conflict, intensifying the forceful interaction between the agent and the patient.

(2) The construction compels the agent and the patient to be linked through resulting behaviors in words and sentences, enhancing the directionality of the action and increasing the overall transitivity and productivity of the clause.

(3) Unlike English three-element causative constructions, Chinese places cognitive emphasis on the resulting state of the patient rather than the process of causation.

Analyzing the constructional meaning of the Ba construction using force dynamics theory can provide a consistent cognitive explanation for unresolved issues pertaining to the Ba construction. Additionally, it establishes a common theoretical foundation for conducting in-depth comparisons of the cognitive models underlying English and Chinese expressions of causative behavior.

The analytic causative structure in English often involves three elements—XYZ, with a typical structure being the English-Chinese causative action structure, in which a manner verb combined with a prepositional phrase expressing place serves as the sub-predicate of the result, such as X caused Y to move to Z. The corresponding Chinese expressions mostly take the form of the Ba construction sentences. In this causative behavior, the patient of the causative motion often undergoes physical displacement or shape transformation. Goldberg (2003) summarized the semantic constraints on verb access in this type of caused-motion construction in English. One crucial constraint is that English verbs used in the caused-motion construction must belong to the hit-class rather than the strike-class. In other words, verbs that allow for this construction should only convey the initiation of the action, without implying any actual impact on the subject. Verbs such as "grind", "slice", "break" do not meet this restriction and thus cannot be used in this construction. For example, in the following example sentences, only 1a conforms to English grammar, and 2a, 3a, and 4a are all problematic.

1a. Sam hit the ball across the field.
1b. 山姆把球打过了这片区域。

Cognitive and Contrastive Analysis of Disease Metaphors in English and Chinese

2a. *Sam strike the ball into the hole.
2b. *山姆把球打中进了洞里。
3a. *Sam break the eggs on the floor.
3b. *山姆把鸡蛋打破在地板上。
4a. *Sam mince the meat onto the chopping board.
4b. *山姆剁碎肉在菜板上。/山姆把肉剁碎在菜板上。

Meanwhile, Goldberg (1995) listed several compensation clauses to mitigate this semantic limitation. Among these clauses, the most significant one pertains to the degree of conventionality in the behavior itself, which is commonly referred to as predictability. Certain verbs, despite not meeting the semantic restrictions of typical causative verbs, can still be used in this construction if the denoted behavior is highly conventional and predictable. For instance,

5a. Grind some black pepper over the salad.
5b. *把一些黑胡椒磨碎,撒在沙拉上。
6a. Break the eggs into the bowl.
6b. *把鸡蛋打到碗里。

Upon examining the Chinese translations of the aforementioned example sentences, it becomes apparent that, after being translated into Chinese, most English causative sentences retain their causative nature. Luo & Zhang (2021), in their article comparing expressions of causing movement events in English and Chinese, refer to them as "causing movement" events. In this book, we adopt this terminology and label the resulting movement event expressed through Chinese words and sentences as the Ba construction sentence. Our focus is limited to the examination of physical displacement of specific objects, excluding any imaginary displacement of abstract entities.

Our inquiry revolves around the fact that while Chinese translation sentence examples 2b and 3b are as unacceptable as their English counterparts, the acceptability of 4b and 5b in Chinese appears relatively high. It is evident that the acceptability of 4b and 5b in Chinese is noticeably higher than that of typical causative sentences, such as 山姆剁碎肉在菜板上,磨碎一些黑胡椒在沙拉上. Consequently, we seek to understand the reasons behind this phenomenon. For

Chapter 5 Social-Cultural Analysis of Differences in Expressing Causes of Diseases in English and Chinese

instance, to what extent can the semantic restrictions proposed by Goldberg for English causative constructions be applied to Chinese causative sentences? Furthermore, what are the semantic restrictions, construction meanings, and cognitive factors influencing these causative sentences? This chapter endeavors to address these questions through an exploration of the force dynamic system theory and a comprehensive analysis of language facts and examples.

Causative behavior holds universal significance, capturing the attention of language typology and comparative linguistics. Within construction grammar, Goldberg (1995a/1995b) delineated the restrictions on verbs used in the English three-element causative action construction, emphasizing that only monomorphic verbs of the "hit" class can enter this construction. For instance, in English, we can say "The boxer hits his opponent to the ground" but cannot say " * The boxer strikes his opponent to the ground". However, it seems that the corresponding Chinese sentence is not bound by this restriction, allowing for the expression 拳击手把对手打到地上. Here, 打 is a single-morpheme verb, 到 serves as the directional preposition indicating the path of motion, and 拳击手把对手打倒在地上 is also acceptable. In the latter case, the verb 打倒 constitutes a verb-particle compound encompassing both the action and the results of the action concerning the patient, while 在 functions as a preposition denoting the location of motion. It is worth noting that directional prepositions such as 到(to) and 进去(go into) are often incompatible, only allowing for the use of place prepositions like "in" to establish the path. Even so, English place prepositions such as "at/on/in" cannot combine with strike verbs to form a complete causative action structure, as exemplified by " * The boxer strikes his opponent on the face/in the eye/on the floor." Consequently, it becomes evident that the semantic restriction for causative verbs outlined by Goldberg (1995a/1995b) for English causative constructions are not entirely applicable to corresponding Chinese causative verb sentences. This section will first review existing literature of causation, and then discuss the semantic restrictions of Chinese Ba construction sentences, along with the constructional meaning of Ba construction. Through the comparative analysis of causative motions in English and Chinese, we aim to gain more insights into the conceptualization of causes in general and causes for disease in English and Chinese.

At the syntactic level, causation can be classified into lexical causation, morphological causation, and analytic causation (Payne, 1997). Huang (2014) built on this classification by categorizing Chinese verb-particle compound words as instances of analytic causative-linked structures, including 打破,剁碎,推倒. However, it is important to note that verb-particle compounds in modern Chinese are originally distinct verbs in ancient Chinese, such as 关闭－阖,粘住－置,据－占领 (Zhang, 2020). These verb-particle compound words exhibit a high degree of cohesion and do not allow for intermediate intervention. Additionally, verb-particle compound words consist of two roots and entail two functional morphemes. Comrie (1989) viewed lexical causation and analytic causation as a continuum, which reveals that in comparison to other causative structure expressions in Chinese, the linking structures composed of verb-particle compounds lean more towards lexical causation.

Simultaneously, the form of the verb sentence aligns more closely with the characteristics of indirect causation within analytic causation, displaying greater syntactic similarities with the three-element analytic causative structure found in English, that is the typical "verb + object + complement". Three-element causative constructions in English usually can only be translated into Chinese sentences involving the use of the Ba construction. For example, "hit the ball across the field" would be translated as 把球打过球场 and cannot be translated as *打球过球场. However, current research on indirect causative analysis in Chinese predominantly focuses on causative sentences composed of compound causative verbs (Huang, 2014), paying relatively little attention to indirect causative behavior expressed through the Ba construction sentences.

There is a possibility of conversion between lexical causation and analytic causation, for example, the English lexical causation "mince". "The butcher minced the beef" can be expressed as "The butcher chopped the beef into paste" with the analytic causation. So the question is "Does this conversion also exist in Chinese?" We believe it is. For example, 屠夫剁碎了牛肉 is caused by the verb 剁碎, which is closer to lexical causation; while the verbal expression 屠夫把牛肉剁碎了 is closer to analytical causation in structure. This kind of analytic verb-oriented sentences that can be derived from lexical-causal conversion is the research focus of this book, without talking about complex sentences with explicit causative verbs, such as "Xiaoli invited Xiaozhang to visit his room", and simple sentences

Chapter 5 Social-Cultural Analysis of Differences in Expressing Causes of Diseases in English and Chinese

with the same predicate verb and non-accusative verb, such as 花瓶碎了 (Hu, 2014).

The specific research scope is limited to the event of the causing behavior with physical displacement; the event includes the actor and the subject, and the subject is displaced by an external force, which is not a spontaneous behavior; the force of the actor is the movement of the subject or the necessary reason for the change, and the force of the agent is in the same direction as the movement of the subject. The object of study is Chinese verbal sentences corresponding to the English-Chinese analytic causative action structure (X causes Y to move to Z). For example, according to Goldberg's four classifications of causative behavior structures (cause-enable, cause-aid, cause-prevent, cause-conditions of satisfaction), in this chapter, we only discuss caused-enable. The causative action sentences with additional conditions are not included, and the scope of the Chinese causative action sentences involved is basically the same as the disposition sentence defined in the grammar of Chinese.

5.2 Social-Cultural Factors for Different Semantic Restraints for Causative Motions

Most studies that focus on the expression of causative syntactic forms believe that causation is not two events, but formed by adding a causer argument (Causer) to the basic clause (Payne, 1997). Huang (2014) believes that if the level of argument increase is extended from the clause to the vocabulary, for example, the increase of functional morphemes in a single vocabulary is also included, or the causative semantics can be summarized as adding arguments at the vocabulary or clause level.

At the semantic level, the causative category is generally regarded as composed of two events, causing and being caused (Comrie, 1989; Song, 2001; Shibatani, 2002). Hu (2014) further put forward the hypothesis of "decomposition of events" that can be discarded, arguing that human beings do not necessarily need the abstract causative predicate when expressing causative meaning, and tried to explain causation by combining syntax and semantics. Goldberg (1995a/1995b) pointed out in construction grammar that some subtle semantic and pragmatic factors play a key role in understanding the constraints of grammatical structures, so he focused on the semantic access restrictions of causative constructions, and regarded causative behavior as a figure of speech that refers to a course of action by source and result states. Ruiz de Mendoza & Usón (2008) further pointed out that the boundaries between the two types of causative constructions that focus on causative actions and results are not clear, but lie on a rhetorical scale. The higher the rhetorical degree, the more result-oriented the expression construction is. Under the framework of event semantics theory, the causative structure is regarded as a different logical combination relationship between two sub-events, emphasizing the semantic generation process of the causative structure and the core role of the causative predicate verb (Wu & Tian, 2018). On the lexical level, starting from lexical semantics, Wang & Wu (2020) disassembled the semantics of causative verbs into three types: the behavioral meaning of X acting on Y, the causative meaning of X making Y a certain state, and the Y means the status of reaching a certain result. Yang (2021) compared the correspondence between the roots and the functional morphemes of causative words in English and Chinese, and found that English causative verbs usually allow one root to multiple functional morphemes, while Chinese allows multiple roots to one functional morpheme case.

Combing the literature, we can see that the latest research on causation structure starts from semantics and focuses on the semantic and syntactic interfaces of causation. However, in view of the complexity of the behavior itself and the diversification of meanings, most of the research is still at the stage of description, failing to analyze more detailed cognitive causes, and unable to provide a convincing general explanation. In terms of the comparison of causative expressions between English and Chinese, domestic studies have investigated the subclassification and valence of verbs in English and Chinese basic causative expressions (Pan & Zhang, 2005), and explored the syntactic and semantic features of English and Chinese classic causative constructions (Chen, 2009), the grammatical metonymy phenomenon of English causative constructions, and the semantic classification and linguistic features of "into V-ing causative constructions" (Zhang, Liu & Liu, 2019), but the research on the similarities and differences of the semantic constraints of English and Chinese in terms of the behavioral construction has not been seen.

Wu & Tian (2018) described the causative meaning of the words and sentences within the formalized event semantics framework, but did not involve the semantic features of the meaning of words and sentences. Wu believes that the Ba construction, which expresses the meaning of causation, emphasizes the change attribute of the causative process and the action behavior that leads to the result. However, this book holds a different point of view, and believes that words and sentences expressing the meaning of disposition don't emphasize the behavior rather than the state and the spatial position that lead to the behavior. Although there are still disputes about whether words and sentences can be classified as causation, it is better to start answering the question of when to use words and sentences. From the perspective of specification to description, the more core question is not when to use it, but "What is the fundamental driving force for using words and sentences?" (Zhang, 2020). If classifying words and sentences as a structure expressing causative meaning in modern Chinese can better explain the fundamental driving force of using words and sentences, then it is advisable to classify words and sentences as causative meanings for the time being.

Not only is there controversy over the division of words and sentences, but there are also different angles of theoretical interpretation of the usage of words and sentences. Cai & Zhang (2017) quoted the explanation of Sybesma (1999) in their article, and believed that the causative light verb V-cause in Chinese causative sentences can be displayed as a Ba sentence merely for the sake of phonetics, but this explanation can not justify why some sentences can only be completed using the Ba structure. For example, 小明把球打进洞 (Xiaoming hit the ball into the hole). Here it is obvious that the Ba sentence cannot be regarded as a display mode of the phonetic morphology of the light verb V-cause.

As a typical causative construction in Chinese, the corresponding subject and argument in the sentence expressing disposition is an agent, an external force with a will. Zhang (2001) proposed that the typical Ba sentence expresses the meaning of causative displacement, and divides the sentence into three types according to the form: the Ba verb-direction construction composed of the main verb and the directional verb, the Ba directional phrase construction, and the Ba directional phrase construction in which directional prepositional phrases such as 过 (through),

Cognitive and Contrastive Analysis of Disease Metaphors in English and Chinese

向 (to) and 朝 (towards) are placed before the verb. According to the classification, this article focuses on the second category, which contains the key information of the path of the preposition list. Zhu (2019) formalized the typical sentence structure as "X + ba Y + VR", where X is the subject and the cause, Y is the object, V is the verb, and R is the verb's complement, object, tense and aspect components, etc. According to this classification, this chapter discusses the situation where R is a preposition with information about the end of the path as a complement, such as "chop the pork on the board" or "push the thief to the ground".

Although some researches have classified and categorized the sentences, the unique semantic restrictions of the verb sentences compared with the general cause have not been fully explained. Words and sentences are traditionally classified as disposition sentences within Chinese grammatical system, so the sentence structure not only requires describing specific behaviors, but also includes the completion of behaviors and performance results. In view of this, some studies have pointed out that because of the high requirements of the result-oriented meaning in the sentence, and the verbs with the embedded resultary meaning in Chinese are mostly verb compound words, or the so-called 动结 verb-conclusion compound words, so the verbs that can enter the verbal sentence must be verbs with concluding meaning. Formal compound words, verbs with mono-syllable and mono-morpheme cannot enter. However, this generalization does not take into account cases where non-verb-conjunctive compounds are followed by a prepositional list path, such as:

小明把球打到屋顶上。
小张把花瓶摔到地上。

The above two example sentences are caused motion lead by causative verbs, but the causative verbs 打 and 打 are both mono-syllable and mono-morpheme verbs, not verb-conjunctive compound words. This shows that the current analysis of the semantic constraints of verb access and subsequent path prepositions in Ba construction verbs is not sufficient, and there are still many unexplained usages of the existing restrictive rules. In addition, as a unique Chinese analytic causative expression, there may be a deeper cognitive reason for the difference between

Chapter 5 Social-Cultural Analysis of Differences in Expressing Causes of Diseases in English and Chinese

English and Chinese causative constructions in terms of the verb access and path prepositions. In view of this, this chapter attempts to explore the impact of semantic changes of causative vocabulary on the form of causative expressions, with special attention paid to the meaning analysis of Chinese verb sentence constructions, the access of verbs and the semantic restrictions of prepositions followed by paths. Besides, we intend to contrast the semantic restrictions in Chinese causative construction with the semantic constraints of the English triple analytic causative construction, and explore the cognitive causes behind the differences.

Goldberg (1995a/1995b) pointed out that the English three-element causative action construction only allows verbs corresponding to a single morpheme, that is, hit-class, while a root corresponds to two morphemes, such as "action + result verbs", that is, strike-class, cannot enter this construction. For example, the following causative construction is ungrammatical: * She filled water into the tub. * He covered the blanket over Mary. The reason is that "fill" and "cover" contain the effect of motion on the caused object, so generally it cannot be followed by a preposition representing the path of motion, that is, it cannot enter the ternary causative behavior construction.

Many verbs in English are verbs with a single root pairing action plus two functional morphemes, such as "strike" and "break". Although causation can be achieved independently, because it is a root pairing two functional morphemes, it cannot enter the causative action that includes the behavior path construction. In contrast, in Chinese, actions and results are often expressed through different morphemes, and the combination of the two action-result verbs, such as "shattering" and "pushing down", to express the meaning of causation. Can the verb-conclusion compound word correspond to two functional morphemes enter the causative action construction? Let's look at the following sets of example sentences:

7a. 小明把花瓶打碎了。
Xiaoming broke the vase.
7b. 小明把花瓶打碎到地上。
* Xiaoming smashed the vase to the ground.
7c. 小明把花瓶打碎在地上。

* Xiaoming smashed the vase on the ground.

8a. 小张把小李推倒了。

Xiaozhang pushed Xiaoli down.

8b. 小张把小李推倒到地上。

* Xiaozhang pushed Xiaoli to the ground.

8c. 小张把小李推倒在地上。

* Xiaozhang pushed Xiaoli to the ground.

9a. 小李把鸡蛋打破了。

Xiaoli broke the egg.

9b. 小李把鸡蛋打破到碗里。

Xiaoli broke the eggs into a bowl.

9c. 小李把鸡蛋打破在碗里。

Xiaoli broke the eggs in a bowl.

It can be seen from the above example sentences that Chinese Ba-causative structure also does not possess a high degree of acceptance for the combination of result-included causative structure with the directional preposition 到 to indicate the path. However, if the directional preposition 到 is replaced by the local preposition 在 (in), the acceptability of the sentence will be significantly improved. At the same time, 7c and 8c are more acceptable than 9c, mainly because the location adverbial guided by 在 is affected by the geometric space characteristics of the following location, that is, the flat ground is a more suitable location for using local preposition 在 that bowl, which is more of a container.

The above analysis shows that the semantic restriction of English causative action constructions exerts less constraint on Chinese Ba construction causative verbs. In the Chinese Ba-causative sentence, even the verbs containing the result of the action can be matched with the preposition to indicate the path for the behavior, and the preposition of place is more acceptable than the preposition of direction. The reason may be related to the emphasis on the initial action and the end point of the behavior in the Chinese Ba construction sentence, which will be analyzed in detail in the next section.

Goldberg (1995a/1995b) proposed a compensation clause for the entry condition of verbs in the English causative action construction, that is, if the

Chapter 5 Social-Cultural Analysis of Differences in Expressing Causes of Diseases in English and Chinese

behavior is highly predictable according to common sense, and the physical displacement of the object can be generally regarded as an incidental behavioral result of the change of physical form, even words with a single root pair and two functional morphemes can enter this construction, such as:

10a. The butcher sliced the salami onto the wax paper.
10b. Joey clumped his potatoes into the middle of his plate.
10c. Joey grated the cheese onto a serving plate.
10d. Sam shredded the papers into the garbage pail.

According to Goldberg, the effect of the verbs in the above sentences are a change in the physical form of the subject, causing the physical displacement of the object is the usual incidental result of the form change, and this incidental displacement is highly predictable, as mentioned above "Sam broke the egg into the bowl". Since a preposition of direction refers to this path with displacement behavior, it can be followed by a preposition. But because this interpretation is based on the conventionality of the causative action, it is affected by the causative scene, so it is difficult to accept the same verb in an uncommon scene, such as * "Sam broke the egg onto the floor".

For Chinese causative verbs involving changes in physical form, is it also possible to allow highly predictable incidental displacement behaviors to be expressed through directional prepositions? Since the explanation is judged based on the conventions in a specific culture, we choose the customary behavior in Chinese culture for analysis.

11a. 李大厨把土豆切到菜板上。
Chef Li cuts the potatoes onto the cutting board.
11b. 李大厨把土豆切片到菜板上。
* Chef Li slices the potatoes onto the cutting board.
12a. 老王把鸡蛋打到碗里。
* Lao Wang cracked the eggs into a bowl.
12b. 老王把鸡蛋打破到碗里。
Lao Wang broke the eggs into the bowl.

The behaviors in the above-mentioned Chinese verbs are highly predictable routines in Chinese culture, but when the "action + result" compound verb is followed by the directional preposition 到, the acceptability of the path is still very low, and it can be seen that predictability, as a supplementary clause for the semantic restriction of English causative action construction verbs, is not applicable to Chinese Ba-causation structure.

Goldberg's semantic restriction emphasizes the decisive and controlling power of the causative verb on the action path of the subject, that is, the physical displacement of the subject is caused and completed by the force of the causative verb. For example,

13a. *He nudged the ball down the incline, unless there are repetitive nudges.
13b. He nudged the golf ball into the hole.

Sentence 13a is unacceptable because "nudge" only induces motion and cannot determine the trajectory of the ball rolling down the slope, in other word, the fact that the ball rolls down the slope is mainly the result of gravity. But sentence 13b is not affected by external force, and the trajectory of the golf ball is completely determined and controlled by the nudge.

14a. 他把球碰下了坡。
He knocked the ball downhill.
14b. 他轻轻一碰,球下了坡。
He makes a light touch and the ball goes downhill.
15a. 他把高尔夫球碰进了洞。
He hit the golf ball in the hole.
15b. 他轻轻一碰,高尔夫球进了洞。
He touched it lightly, and the golf ball went into the hole.

Judging from the Chinese translations of the above sentences, although Sentences 14a and 15a are more in line with the Chinese expression habits, Sentences 14b and 15b are also acceptable in Chinese. It can be seen that this semantic restriction does not apply to Chinese words and verbs either. For another example, 小明把球推下了斜坡 (Xiaoming pushed the ball down the slope), the verb 推 (push) in this sentence can be understood as a non-sustained and nonrepeatable initial force, which is not the only dominant force of the behavior path, and cannot completely control the path trajectory, but this sentence in Chinese is perfectly acceptable. The corresponding English sentence "He pushed the ball down the slope" can only be interpreted as the actor has been pushing the ball down the slope all along the path; it cannot be understood as just "nudged the ball", and then the ball rolled down by itself. This is the result of restricting the semantics of the verb "push" in the behavioral construction. So how does Chinese specifically express the situation that the actor and the ball go downhill together? At this time, the expression that is more in line with the Chinese expression habit is 他推着球下了坡 (He went down the hill pushing the ball). In the sentence an aspect marker 着 is added.

Through the comparative analysis of causative expressions in English and Chinese, we found that the division of causative action constructions in English is affected by the agent's decisiveness and control over the process of the subject's movement, and only those with strong decisiveness and control over the behavior process can enter the causative action construction. However, this semantic limitation does not apply to the use of Chinese Ba-causation construction, which emphasizes the starting force and the end point, and does not highlight the agent's control over the behavior process of the recipient. This conclusion can also better explain why Sentences 14a and 15a above are more in line with Chinese expression habits than Sentences 14b and 15b. Therefore, it can be summarized that whether Chinese verbs in the Ba construction can be followed by a locational or directional preposition is not subject to the semantic restriction of the complete control clause as in English causative construction.

5.3 Force Dynamic Analysis of Causative Motions

Cultural conceptualization can be seen as larger allegorical complexes, where metaphors can serve as metonymic references to an allegorical complex. This reference to the allegorical complex operates like a set of conceptually related schemas. In other words, what's been activated is a group of frameworks, constructions or schema, which consists of a series of concepts, ideas and events.

When one node of this giant network is triggered, the whole "net" will become activated, and those highlighted nodes will emerge from the network to form the functioning image schema in the process of meaning construal. For example, when we say we are eating out today, the whole dining in a restaurant event frame will be activated. The same logic also applies to the use of metaphor, when we compare the cause of disease to the "root", the whole "tree" image will appear in our brain to make sure the "Root" metaphor works. This is not just a single metaphor, but a complex of metaphors that are adopted as a system of related conceptualization, which can serve to activate scripts and simulations, inform behavior, increase performativity in blended spaces or even shape identity.

Compared with the Chinese causative action sentences with general word order, the lexical causative sentence can relax the restriction of the causative structure on the action followed by the prepositional phrase, that is, the general causative sentence can be transformed into lexical causative. In other words, compared with the Chinese verb-resultative construction, the lexical structure of the verb sentence has a stronger transitivity in the syntax. From this, it can be inferred that the sentence structure itself is meaningful. Verbs are viewed as a construction (Fillmore, 1988; Goldberg, 1995a/1995b).

According to the LCM (Lexical Construction Model) theory, the process of constructing form and meaning is subject to internal and external restrictions. The external restriction refers to the process of adapting the meaning of words to the meaning of the construction, that is, the construction has the function of "coercion", and the related elements can impose on another linguistic configuration and cause that configuration to transform (Pustejovsjy, 1993), and transformations are cognitive in nature (Ruiz de Mendoza & Usón, 2008). Force dynamics, as the main theoretical system to explain semantics from the perspective of cognition, has theoretical explanatory power for the analysis of construction meaning construction. The above analysis of the Ba construction causative sentence shows that the verbs in the Ba construction causative sentences are not limited by the single-morpheme verbs in the English causative action structure, and can be followed by the path of the preposition table. The trajectory of the movement has complete determination and control. In the following text, we will combine the force-dynamic theory to explain the cognitive motivation of the causative

Chapter 5 Social-Cultural Analysis of Differences in Expressing Causes of Diseases in English and Chinese

construction, and compare the Chinese Ba causative construction with the English causative action construction. In this way, we can better understand the English and Chinese conceptualization of the causative motion, and gain deeper insights of the cognition of causes for disease, as well as the accompanying social-cultural elements.

Sentences expressing dynamic patterns can choose combinations of different factors to express their referents without mentioning the rest. That is, some factors are selected to refer to the whole force dynamic mode. Generally speaking, factors that appear clearly, earlier, or at a higher character level are more foreground and more likely to attract attention. Compared with the causative action sentences in natural order, the confrontation between the anti-body force and the main force in the word causative verb sentence is strengthened. For example, "The child pushes the ball down the hill" is a causative action sentence of natural order, which means that the child and the ball go down the hill together. During this action, the acting force must continue throughout the entire action process. The force conflict is not enough to support the subject (the ball) to complete the trajectory downhill driven by the initial force. The corresponding sentence "The child pushes the ball down the hill" can be understood as "The child did not go down the hill", and the child only exerted an external force on the subject (the ball) as the agent. The reason why the sentence can mean that the ball goes down the hill but the child does not go down the hill can be interpreted from the perspective of force dynamics. The fact is that the construction of the word strengthens the force confrontation between the agent and the recipient, and strengthens the continuity of the causative force and control. Gawron (1986) used a double predicate-verb predicate and a prepositional predicate to explain the causative action construction in English, and believed that the second preposition assists the verb predicate in explaining the action of the agent on the subject at the pragmatic level. Using words to enhance the force conflicts in verbal sentence constructions and coercing prepositions of place into directional interpretations that express behavioral trajectories are similar to the functions of the second predicate of prepositions in English, which can assist verbs and predicates to achieve the strengthening of force.

The argument that the Ba construction can strengthen the subject-object confrontation can also be confirmed from the types of verbs that the structure

Cognitive and Contrastive Analysis of Disease Metaphors in English and Chinese

allows. It can be found that non-ergative verbs that do not highlight action force cannot enter the Ba causative construction verb sentence that contains three elements, such as 张三把李四哭得很伤心（*Zhang San makes Li Si cry badly.）(three-element, non-ergative)/把我笑傻了（*This made me laugh as an idiot)/这把我笑惨了（*This made me laugh so badly）. All of these three Chinese Ba sentences are ungrammatical. Meanwhile, non-accusative verbs that highlight action force can be used in verb sentences, for example, 这酒把张三醉得站不起来（Zhang San was so drunk that he couldn't stand up）(ternary non-accusative case). One possible explanation is that the verbs "laugh" and "cry" have not imposed any force on the subject that is against the subject's will, that is, the force confrontation is not obvious, which does not match the meaning of the Ba construction, thus the verb can not enter the Ba causative construction. In other words, only verbs that highlight the constructory external force can enter the Ba construction, which also confirms the argument that the Ba causative construction strengthens the force confrontation of the word. More example sentences are as follows,

16a. 李厨把鱼摔死在地上。

*Chef Li smashed the fish dead on the ground.

16b. 李厨摔了好几次，终于把一条活蹦乱跳的鱼摔死在地上。

Smashing the fish several times, Chef Li finally managed to smash the fish dead on the ground.

17a. 李厨把猪肉剁碎在板子上。

*Chef Li minced the pork onto the chopping board.

17b. 细细地剁了好久，李厨把猪肉都剁碎在板子上。

*Chopping the pork for quite a while, Chef Li minced all the pork onto the chopping board.

The above example sentences are all grammatical in Chinese, but the corresponding English sentences are inappropriate. Since both "smash" and "mince" include the influence on the patient, they cannot be allowed into the English XYZ causative action construction (Goldberg, 1995a/1995b). At the same time, compared with Sentences 16a and 17a, the Chinese example sentences 16b and 17b have a higher degree of acceptance, and the reason can also be

Chapter 5 Social-Cultural Analysis of Differences in Expressing Causes of Diseases in English and Chinese

explained consistently by the previous argument that the Ba construction strengthens the confrontation between the agent and the patient. The repeated use of bounded and non-sustainable verbs can enhance the strength of force confrontation between the agent force and the force from the patient. It is due to the repeated use of verbs such as 摔 (smash) and 剁 (cut), that the confrontation force between the agent and recipient is enhanced. Thus, the increased confrontation with force makes the meaning of the context more consistent with the meaning of the construction of the Ba sentence, leading to a higher degree of acceptability.

The Ba construction can highlight the characteristics of force confrontation, which can also be further confirmed by the answers to the typical interrogative sentences of the Ba sentence, for example, 小张把小明怎么样了？（What did Xiaozhang do to Xiaoming?）, the possible answers to the Chinese question are listed as follows：

18a.　*小张把小明换了件新衣服。
　*Xiaozhang changed Xiaoming into a new dress.
18b.　*小张把小明抱了抱。
　*Xiaozhang hugged Xiaoming.
19a.　小张把小明打了一顿。
　Xiaozhang beat Xiaoming up.
19b.　小张把小明赶出了门。
　Xiaozhang kicked Xiaoming out of the house.

The reason why Sentences 18a and 18b are unacceptable is not because of the problem of syntactic structure, but because there is no force confrontation between the agent and the patient, which is inconsistent with the meaning of the Ba construction that increases the confrontation force of the sentences, so it can not enter the Ba-construction sentence. The corresponding sentences 19a and 19b are completely acceptable, because it can be foreseen that Xiaoming does not want to be beaten, nor does he want to be kicked out of the house, so there is a confrontation force between the agent and the recipient; therefore, the sentences are acceptable.

According to the parameters for evaluating transitivity of clauses, it can be concluded that the Ba-construction causative sentence is a clause with strong transitivity if we continue to ask what is the specific reason for the strong transitivity. Hopper and Tompson believe that based on the theory of force dynamics, three reasons can be summarized. The first is that the words lexicalize the force confrontation between the agent and the recipient, which improves the degree of action and agency from structural sense, and enhances the initial force. This point has been demonstrated in detail in the previous sections. Secondly, the predicate verb and the following location word (noun or prepositional phrase) are coerced into an action link by the Ba-causative construction, and the strengthened link increases the directionality of the action itself, which is beneficial to the continuation of the causative force. Thirdly, the cognitive focus of words and sentences is on the result of the event, because the result of the event is foregrounded, thus allowing a more diversified expressions of the results. Diversified expressions also improve the acceptability of prepositional phrases followed by paths and locations, and the reasons for this will be discussed in the following sections.

According to the theory of force dynamics, the enhancement of force confrontation means that the entire resulting behavior has greater tension, which is manifested as a clearer path to the realization of the force dynamic mode on the psychological level, and stronger transitivity in the form of language expression. In a word, the strength of the force resistance of the causative action is directly proportional to the transitivity of sentence. The reason why the transitivity of the causative action sentence is higher than that of the general causative action sentence is that the use of the word Ba strengthens the resistance force. For example, the example sentences 16a, 16b, 17a and 17b above are allowed to be followed by prepositional phrases to indicate the end point of the subject's movement trajectory only in the Ba-causative construction, such as 李厨把鱼摔在地上（Chef Li smashed the fish to the ground）/李厨把猪肉剁碎在菜板上（*Chef Li minced the pork on the cutting board）, while the same structure can not be accepted in general causative action sentence without the Ba construction, for example, 李厨摔(死)鱼在地上（*Chef Li threw dead fish on the ground）/李厨剁碎猪肉在菜板上（*Chef Li chopped pork on the cutting board）, both cannot be accepted.

The example sentences given above are all example sentences with explicit agent. There is another Ba-construction that omits agent, such as 把小明打倒

Chapter 5   Social-Cultural Analysis of Differences in Expressing Causes of Diseases in English and Chinese

(knock down Xiaoming), 把菜洗净 (wash the vegetables), and 把肉剁碎 (chop the meat). Then, can the sentences that omit the agent be followed by a prepositional structure to indicate the path of the action?

20a. 小张把小明打倒。
Xiaozhang beat Xiaoming down.
20b. 小张把小明打倒在地上。
Xiaozhang knocked Xiaoming to the ground.
20c. 把小明打倒在地上。
Knock Xiaoming to the ground.

Through comparison, it is found that the acceptability of Sentence 20c in Chinese is significantly lower than that of Sentence 20b. That is to say, the sentence omitting the agent often cannot be followed by a preposition, and the transitivity of the sentence is weakened. But Sentence 20b, which does not omit the agent, can be followed by a preposition. This phenomenon can further confirm the argument that force confrontation is positively correlated with transitivity. When both the agent and the patient are clearly mentioned, both are foregrounded, which can present a complete confrontation, resulting in strong transitivity, so it can be followed by location or directional preposition to indicate the action path. However, in Sentence 20c, due to the lack of agent, the force confrontation can not be manifested, and the transitivity of the sentence is weakened, so the acceptability of the following preposition is low.

From the perspective of syntactic structure, adding the functional connective Ba between the agent and the recipient can leave more slots to describe the concretization of the causative force elements continuously. The improved structure can increase the expansion potentiality of Chinese sentence. Moreover, cross-lingual evidence shows that it is a common grammatical phenomenon that adding identification marks to the object can give more freedom to the word order of the sentence (Luo, 2021). Object markers whose positions change more freely have a positive effect on the strengthening of sentence transitivity. In addition, according to the viewpoint that compactness is inversely correlated to productivity and transitivity (Shibatani & Pardeshi, 2002), given that the compactness of verb sentences is lower than that of Chinese verb-resultative vocabulary, its productivity

Cognitive and Contrastive Analysis of Disease Metaphors in English and Chinese

is correspondingly higher than direct. Due to its lexical nature, it can be followed not only by adjectives, but also by the prepositional phrase "成（form）+ N" and the prepositional adverbial "在（at）+ location", for example,

Verb-conjugated lexical causes:

21a. 小明摔碎了花瓶。
Xiaoming broke the vase.
21b. 小明摔(碎)了花瓶个稀巴烂。
* Xiaoming smashed (broke) the vase to pieces.
21c. * 小明摔(碎)了花瓶成碎片。
* Xiaoming smashed (broke) the vase into pieces.
21d. * 小明摔碎花瓶在地上。
* Xiaoming smashed the vase on the ground.

Ba-causative construction:

22a. 小明把花瓶摔碎了。
Xiaoming broke the vase.
22b. 小明把花瓶摔了个稀巴烂。
Xiaoming smashed the vase to pieces.
22c. 小明把花瓶摔成了碎片。
Xiaoming broke the vase into pieces.
22d. 小明摔碎花瓶在地上。
Xiaoming smashed the vase on the ground.

The above example sentences further prove that the verb sentence with Ba construction has higher productivity and transitivity than the causative sentence with the lexical cause, and combined with the explanation of the dynamic theory of power and the examples of language facts, it can be deduced that the word Ba strengthens the force resistance. The overall causative force of a sentence is the cognitive motivation to improve the transitivity and productivity of causative sentences.

In English causative action sentences, the bimorphic verbs, such as "break" and "smash", which correspond to the Chinese verb-resultative prase like 摔破 and

Chapter 5 Social-Cultural Analysis of Differences in Expressing Causes of Diseases in English and Chinese

摔碎, cannot be followed by other modifiers, for example, " * Xiaoming broke the vase into pieces", " * Xiaoming broke the vase onto the floor", neither of them conforms to the English habits of expression. Fillmore (1988) described the prepositional phrase in the causative action construction that indicates the position of the subject space in this way, taking "The dog put the bone in the kennel" as an example, what is finally positioned in the kennel is not any object, state or an event, but the end point of the action "to put" that completes the verb's argument role goal. Fillmore's description of the causative construction followed by a space prepositional phrase shows that English emphasizes the action process information when expressing the causative action. The focus of information is on the causative verb, while the spatial position of the subject is only to maintain the integrity of the action process. However, the expression of the causative event in Chinese is quite different from that in English. It focuses on the change and displacement of the subject under the force of the agent, and can simultaneously express the result state and spatial position of the patient. The force confrontation between the agent and the patient and the result state of the patient are the core semantic elements, which is both the cognitive focus and the foregrounded information in the force dynamic sequence.

According to the stage division of the force dynamic sequence, while the Ba-causative construction can strengthen the force confrontation, the cognitive focus of Ba sentence can only focus on the results that have happened or not happened, but not on the behavior process. For example,

23a. 小张把小明请进屋。

Xiaozhang invites Xiaoming into the house. (the connotate meaning in Chinese Ba sentence is: Xiaoming entered the house, which is not the case in the English translation)

23b. 小张没把小明请进屋。

Xiaozhang did not invite Xiaoming into the house. (meaning: Xiaoming did not enter the house)

24a. 小张请小明进屋。

Xiaozhang invites Xiaoming into the house. (From this Chinese sentence whether Xiaoming entered the house or not is not clear.)

24b. 小张没请小明进屋。

Xiaozhang did not invite Xiaoming into the house. (Whether Xiaoming entered the house is not clear.)

Whether in terms of the stage in force dynamic sequences, it can be seen from the above example sentences that in Sentences 23a and 23b, the highlighted is the result part, that is, "whether Xiaoming entered the house", and its cognitive focus is the result state of the subject, which is specifically expressed as the end point of the subject's trajectory spatial location. In contrast, in Sentences 24a and 24b, the attention is distributed in the initial stage of the causative action, that is, the action "invite", the attention window appears earlier, and the uncertain result is backgrounded.

Generally, causative action sentences cannot support the follow-up path and end point information because the attention window is the action itself rather than the result state of the subject, such as *李厨打破鸡蛋在碗里 (Chef Li broke the egg in the bowl), where 打破 (break) is the foregrounded initial action. The broken egg as the result state of the patient is a the non-foregrounded secondary result, and the attention window is not in the result position; therefore, the sentence does not support prepositional path information, and the sentence does not conform to the Chinese expression habits. However, in Chinese Ba sentence, the word Ba appears before the action. Through lexicalizing force confrontation, Ba structure strengthens the external force that continues the attention to the end of the behavior path, and at the same time, its construction link meaning coerces the attention to move back to the result stage of the force dynamic sequence, so the acceptability of 李厨把鸡蛋打破在碗里 is significantly higher than 李厨打破鸡蛋在碗里. That is to say, Ba structure's emphasis on the result state of the partient is the inevitable result of the strengthened force confrontation and the in creased transitivity of the sentence, which is further reflected in that Ba sentence allows more information about the result state of the patient.

The above claim can also be argued from another perspective. It is exactly because that the cognitive focus of Chinese words and sentences is on the result of the action, which makes it impossible to express the causative action itself without mentioning the result of action. This can be confirmed from the fact that the

Chapter 5 Social-Cultural Analysis of Differences in Expressing Causes of Diseases in English and Chinese

following Chinese words and sentences cannot simply express wishes, orders or requests. There are obvious differences with the English causative action construction. Verbs expressing wishes, orders, requests, etc. in English can express situations where the result is unknown, while Chinese Ba-causative verbal sentence cannot, such as:

25a. Sam ordered him out of the house. (Goldberg, 2003: 161)
山姆命令他出去。(Whether the action of going out is completed is unknown)
*山姆把他命令了出去。

25b. Sam asked him into the room. (Goldberg, 2003: 161)
山姆叫他进房间。(whether entered unknown)
山姆把他叫进房间。(It means that the person has already entered the room, which does not match the aspectual meaning of the English sentence)

25c. Sam beckoned him into the room. (Goldberg, 2003: 161)
山姆求他进房间。(whether entered unknown)
山姆把他求进房间。(indicating that the person has entered the room, which does not match the aspectual meaning of the English sentence)

It can be seen from the above example sentences that Chinese Ba sentence cannot express the situation where the result of the action is unknown. The reason still goes to the above explanation within the force dynamic sequence. Due to the fact that the Ba construction foregrounds the resultative stage of the sequence, so the sentence does not allow to the cognitive focus to be in the unknown state. At the same time, the above-mentioned example sentences expressing intentions also show that the Ba construction has the characteristics of "coercing" the verb into the meaning of the result. Even for the behavior without a definite result, once it enters the Ba construction, it is "coerced" to a structure which has definite behavior result as the default-meaning.

In addition, Chinese is a topic-oriented language, and the focus of information in a sentence is mostly at the end of the sentence. In terms of word order, the prepositional phrase in the causative action structure of the Chinese Ba sentence can only be placed at the end of the sentence, while the position of the prepositional phrase in the English causative action construction is more flexible, which can be either at the beginning or at the end of the sentence. As in the following example sentences 26 and 27, this reflects that the spatial orientation of the attention window of the Ba sentence in the force dynamic sequence stage is relatively stable, and it is fixed in the behavior result stage, so the information that represents the behavior path and the outcome state of the subject can only appear at the end of the sentence, and cannot be transferred to the beginning of the sentence. In English, the causative action construction focuses on the action itself and the process, and the attention window moves with the causative force, without emphasizing the stability of the end point of the action path. Therefore, the position of the prepositional phrase expressing the action path in the sentence is relatively flexible.

26. Into the goal, John kicked the ball.
﹡进球门,约翰把球踢。
27. Over the fence, Sam spray the paint.
﹡满栅栏,山姆把漆喷。

Chinese Ba sentences share similar expression form with English resultative constructions (resultative construction), such as "He hammered the iron flat", the corresponding Chinese Ba sentence is 他把铁打平了, and the word order is basically the same. But unlike the causative action construction, the English result construction is generally considered as a new logical structure in which the focus is on the point of accomplishment. However, in Chinese, the Ba sentence covers the situation where the agent causes the patient to undergo a physical displacement or state change, shift, or deform. English grammar sets a clear separating line between the change of location and the change of state, divides and conquers, expressing the causative behavior of physical displacement using the three-element causative behavior construction of X caused Y move to Z, while expressing the physical state change of the subject using the result construction, the focus albeit both lay on the action behavior, the former uses the physical displacement of the event to mark the completion of action, and the latter takes the change of the physical state of object as the node of the completion of action. In a word, the cognition focus of the Chinese Ba construction verb sentence is on the result of action; while the focus of the English causative action construction is on the action itself, focusing on the beginning and end of the movement process or the movement path.

From the perspective of the force dynamic model, the tension of the causative motion structure comes from the confrontation between the agent force and the force of the patient or recipient, and whether the causative result can be followed by a path preposition is related to the concretization of the elements of the force dynamic model. English embodies the specificity of the pattern elements of force dynamics and emphasizes the directionality of action, while Chinese is better at describing the result state of the subject under the action of force in detail. In terms of vocabulary, English possesses more directional prepositional phrases with morpheme verbs, such as "Pat sprayed the paint toward the window / over the fence / through the woods", where "toward", "over" and "through" all express the direction and trajectory of the force extension movement. Meanwhile, the corresponding Chinese translation is 帕特把油漆喷到窗户上/喷满栅栏/喷满木板, among which only 喷到 is "a verb + directional preposition". Although the preposition 到 (to) also indicates directionality, which is the trajectory, more prominent is the spatial location of the end point of the movement rather than the movement process. The other two path prepositions in English are transformed into "verb + adjective": 喷满 is used to express the result state of the patient. In general, Chinese has relatively fewer directional prepositional phrases, but at the same time, the presentation of causative actions is less restricted by verbs, and can be more flexibly distributed in different positions of the sentence and presented in structural forms with different degrees of compactness (Ji, Hendricks & Hickmann, 2011).

5.4 Summary of the Analysis of Causation and Its Implication in Understanding Causes for Disease in English and Chinese

This section attempts to summarize the unique semantic access restrictions of Chinese Ba causative construction sentences compared with English ternary causative-motion structures, and combines the force dynamics theory to explain the constructional meaning of Ba construction sentences from a cognitive perspective. The analysis found that the semantic restriction criteria applicable to English causative motion constructions are not fully applicable to Chinese Ba sentences. For example, in terms of whether the causative action can be followed by a prepositional phrase to indicate the end point of the subject displacement, Chinese Ba causative sentences are compatible with bilingual morpheme verbs, while English only allows single-morpheme hit-class verbs. Besides, English only allows verbs that have absolute and complete control over the movement trajectory of the subject to enter the X caused Y move to Z construction, while there is no such restriction on the verbs that enter Chinese Ba construction.

Although Chinese Ba construction is not restricted by the semantic rules in causative action constructions in English, Ba causative constructions have requirements for the intensity level of the confrontation force implied by the verbs and the prepositions that express the end point of the physical displacement of the patient or recipient. Based on the force dynamics theory, this chapter has proposed a cognitive interpretation of the construction meaning of the Ba sentence, and has deduced three theoretical hypotheses: first, Chinese Ba causative construction strengthens the force confrontation between the agent and the recipient; second, the construction increases the transitivity of the sentence; third, the Ba construction foregrounds the resultortive state of the caused motion. The above theoretical hypotheses can provide a possible consistent explanation for the remaining controvertial questions in the study of Chinese Ba sentences.

Question 1: Research on the relationship between two Chinese causative sentences lead by 使(make) and sentence lead by 把(make), such as the sentence 王玮的态度使刘强把提着的心放了下来(Wang Wei's attitude made Liu Qiang put his heart down), The question is why we can only embed the Ba-structure in the shi-structure, but not vice versa? Wu and Tian's (2018) answer to the above question is that the argument in the shi-structure is the cause, and the argument in the Ba structure is the external force, we can put the cause in front of the external force, but not the other way around. This explanation is not satisfactory. There is no fixed logical relationship between the external force and the cause. The external force can be the cause, and the cause can also be the external force. According to the analysis of force dynamics in the above-mentioned Ba construction sentences, the author believes that the reason why Ba constructions can be embedded in shi-

constructions is that the restriction of force resistance between the agent and the recipient is that shi-structure is low. In other words, the range of force confrontation intensity of shi-construction is greater than the range of force confrontation of Ba-construction, so the Ba structure can be included in the shi-structure, but not vice versa.

Question 2: Why can bare verb sentences be allowed in Chinese Ba sentence? From the perspective of construction meaning, coercion only occurs in connection. Prepositional phrases that do not indicate direction can be allowed in the caused-motion construction, and the construction gives directional interpretation to the locational preposition through "accomodation" and "coercion" (Croft, 1991; Pustejovsky, 1993; Talmy, 2000). As a causative action construction, Chinese Ba construction coerces the predicate verb and the following location word (noun or prepositional phrase) into an action link, and the strengthened link increases the directionality of the causative action itself. At the same time, because "Ba" lexicalizes the force conflict or confrontation force between the agent and the patient/recipient, the causative force has a stronger influence on the main participants involved in the causative behavior, including both the agent and the patient. And the enhancement of action directionality and action force increases the definiteness of the whole sentence. Based on the improved definiteness of the whole sentence, the vacancy of the subject does not affect the realization of the sentence meaning, leading to a higher acceptability of bare verb sentence in Chinese Ba construction.

Question 3: Why is the Ba causative construction more flexible, transitive and productive? Consistent with the results of the English-Chinese causative comparison experiment conducted by Ji, Hendriks & Hickmann (2011), the expression of the result in Chinese causative sentences can be more diversified, and the predicates can be expressed using structures of different density. For example, it can use more compact lexical causation like V1 + V2, and the causative structure can also be realized through the geographical location of the patient using prepositional phrases, especially the adverbial of location, so as to refer to the state of the causative result, compensating the sentence structural density with productivity. The Ba sentence in Chinese is a low-density causative action expression, in which the word Ba lexicalizes the force conflict between the agent and the recipient, and strengthens the force confrontation, while leaving room for the expression of the causative action and result in the syntactic structure a more complete space in form. The strengthened force confrontation provides the initial force for the extension of the causative meaning, and the meaning of the construction of the verb sentence strengthens the directionality of the entire action link, and the meaning of the verb sentence causes the meaning to pay close attention to the result state of the subject as a sentence. The strong transitivity of the sentence lays a cognitive foundation, so the use of words to make the verb sentence is relatively general, so that the action sentence has higher transitivity and productivity.

Question 4: Both English and Chinese are defined as satellite framework languages by Talmy (2000), yet is there a difference in the distance and control of the "satellite"? The cognitive interpretation of Chinese Ba construction also has new theoretical implications for the type dichotomy of verb-frame language and satellite-frame language given by Talmy. Tamly (2000) divided languages into verb-framed language and satellite-framed language according to the different ways of expressing the behavior path. The former is that verb implies the behavior path, and the latter expresses the meaning of the behavior path by satellite words. According to Tamly's classification, both English and Chinese are satellite-frame languages, and the path of behavior is not implied in the semantics of the verb, but is represented by satellite words. In English "A bird flew across the river", the verb "fly" expresses the action itself and the way, across the expression "path". The same is true for the Chinese 小鸟飞过河流 (Birds fly over the river).

Through the analysis of the meaning of the construction of the verb sentence in Chinese, we find that Chinese has more prominent characteristics of satellite-frame language compared with English. There are bimorpheme causative verbs in English, such as "break/smash". The semantics of verbs include both the emission of action and the effect on subject, and the semantics indirectly imply the virtual movement path of action. However, whether the causative verb in Chinese is the lexical causation of the verb-resultative compound word, such as 打倒 (knock down)/打破(break)/打碎(shatter), or the Ba-causative construction 把……打(倒/破/碎)在……上, the initial action verb is 打, and the result affected by the event is represented by a separate Chinese character 倒/破/碎, the movement path is referred to by the prepositional phrase of place after the action 在……上(above). From this point of view, although both English and Chinese are roughly classified into the satellite-framework language, there are still differences in the distance the verb "releases" the "satellite". As far as English and Chinese causative action sentences are concerned, the distance between the "satellites" and the main action in Chinese language is bigger than that in English.

The three theoretical hypotheses of the Chinese Ba sentence and verb sentences based on the theoretical framework of the force dynamics theory can provide a consistent explanation based on cognition for some remaining problems in the study of Ba causative construction sentence, but whether the explanation is universal still needs more investigation. The follow-up research should use the corpus to further verify the explanatory power of the three theoretical hypotheses, and carry out linguistic typology research on the expression forms of causing behaviors, and investigate the extent to which the dynamic interpretation of words and verb sentences has universal explanatory power.

Relational process describes the process type of the logical relationship between entities. He, Wang & Lü (2019) divided it into six sub processes, namely, attributive process, identifying process, locational process, directional process, possessive process and correlational process. There are generally two actors in the relational process.

Attributive process describes some characteristics and attributes of the entity. The two participants of the process are labeled as Carrier and Attribute.

Identifying process reflects the identification relationship between the two participants. Token and value take on the two roles of this process.

Locational process describes the position of the entity in time or space, and the two participants of the process are Carrier and Location.

Directional process describes the state of the entity extending statically to a certain direction. The participants of the process include Source, Path and Destination.

Possessive process describes the ownership relationship between one entity and another, and the two participants of the process are Possessor and Possessed.

Correlational process represents the relevance between two entities, and the two participants of the process are named Correlator 1 and Correlator 2. Based on the relational process division, combined with our quantative and qualitative analysis of disease metaphors in English and Chinese, we have come into conclusions about the similarities and differences between English and Chinese. Let us start with the differences. The first overall cognitive difference in the conceptualization of disease between English and Chinese is that time is a dominant domain in viewing disease in English, while Space is a dominant domain in perceiving disease in Chinese. The detailed argumentation in favor of this claim has already been presented in Chapter 3 through the comparison of "Root" metaphors in English and Chinese. Here we will simply summarize the differences based on the division of relational processes. Among the above processes, locational and possessive processes are more closely related to space-oriented thinking, for one has to activate space domain in order to learn about the location of an item. And the sensory illustration of "possession" is that item A is "held" by subject B, also heavily relying on space-oriented thinking.

Since we argue in the most abstract level that Chinese relies more on space domain in conceptualizing diseases, then naturally possessive and locational processes would be more frequently used in the words and expressions for illness. Then when we look at the most frequent collocates for Chinese character 病, it turns out that the most common expression 有病 (have disease) is indeed highlighting a possessive relationship between the patient and the illness. Specifically, the corpus analysis of related expressions for 病 in Chinese has shown that the verb 有 is the most frequent collocate for 病. The expression 有病 is so widely used that its pragmatic meaning has expanded and can refer to any abnormal social behavior of any individual. Besides, the word 有病 is also a mild curse word to refer to people that are irritating and annoying.

The emphasis on locational process is vividly displayed in the favored usage of 病根 in Chinese. The fact that the composition of the compound word 病根 does not require any preposition suggests that Chinese prefer to use locational relationship when it is available. The formation of 病根 is based on the analogy between the locational proximity between 根 and 树, and that between "cause" and

Chapter 5 Social-Cultural Analysis of Differences in Expressing Causes of Diseases in English and Chinese

"disease". Similar examples can also be found in compound words like 病源, which is mapping the spatial proximity between 源头 (origin) and 河流 (river) to the relationship between "cause" and "disease". Space-oriented locational process takes a dominant position when describing the relationship between "cause" and "disease".

On the contrary, we argue that English depends more on time domain in the conceptualization of disease. And the representative processes would be attributive and directional, both of which are more dynamic and are featured by a clear direction. Attributive process implicates the central object and the characteristics that can be attributed to the described object, in which the cognitive scanning always starts with a particular feature and ends with the target. The corpus searching results also support this argument. The most frequent expression related to "illness" is the adjective form "ill", such as "One is ill", or "One fell ill". In both cases, "ill" is a characteristic that is applied to depict the state of being "ill". It is a clear attributive process in play. Besides, the use of verb "is" and "fell" is indicating a directional process with its beginning, path and destination. In this case, the event starts with a healthy subject, the path is denoted with the verb "is" or "fell", and then the destination is "ill".

The directional process can be found in the most widely used disease metaphor involving part of the plant, that is, "the root of disease", the formation of the phrase depends on the attributive process and directional process. The use of preposition "of" indicates an attributive process, in which "root" is attributed to "disease" through the preposition "of". Meanwhile, the reason that this metaphor can be rendered feasible goes to the similarity in directional process, that is, the process of root growing into a tree is similar to the process that cause leading to the disease. It can be seen that both attributive process and directional process highlight the cognitive scanning that moves from one point to another, which is in line with our argument that English conceptualization of illness relies more on time domain.

The second difference between the perception of illness between English and Chinese is based on the afore mentioned divergence in spatial-temporal cognition. To support the argument that Chinese people tend to objectify illness and focus on its consequences, while English people are more process-oriented and emphasize the illness as a process, we can look at additional evidence from various sources.

Here are a few examples: as for the perceptual differences of illness between Chinese and English, we believe that Chinese people tend to objectify illness, and pay more attention to the consequences of having the illness, while English people are more process-oriented, under the influence of English language, which is time-oriented. Their conceptualization of illness also focuses more on illness as a process. Since the attention is mainly paid to the process, the possible consequences of illness is less emphasized compared with that in Chinese. Chinese culture places strong emphasis on harmony and balance, and illness is often seen as a disruption to this balance. Chinese medicine and traditional beliefs focus on restoring harmony and addressing the consequences of illness. In contrast, English-speaking cultures may have a different cultural understanding of illness, where the focus is more on the process of diagnosing, treating, and managing the illness.

Analyzing the linguistic features of Chinese and English related to illness can provide further evidence. Chinese language has rich vocabulary and expressions related to the consequences and effects of illness, such as 后果 (consequence), 影响 (impact), and 症状 (symptom). On the other hand, English language may have more terms and expressions focused on the process of illness, such as "diagnosis", "treatment", and "recovery". Analyzing medical discourse in Chinese and English can shed light on how illness is conceptualized and discussed. Chinese medical texts and discussions may emphasize the consequences and effects of illness on the body, mind, and overall well-being. In contrast, English medical discourse may focus more on the processes involved in diagnosis, treatment plans, and the progression of illness. Conducting cross-cultural studies comparing Chinese and English speakers' perceptions and attitudes towards illness can provide empirical evidence. These studies can explore participants' beliefs, perceptions, and responses to illness-related scenarios, interviews, or questionnaires, and identify any differences in how they objectify illness or focus on the process.

By examining these sources of evidence, we can gain a deeper understanding of the perceptual differences of illness or disease between Chinese and English speakers, supporting the argument that Chinese tends to objectify disease and focus on consequences, while English tends to be more process-oriented in its conceptualization of disease. Chinese culture values collectivism, harmony, and

Chapter 5 Social-Cultural Analysis of Differences in Expressing Causes of Diseases in English and Chinese

the well-being of the community. Thus disease is often viewed as a disruption to the collective harmony, and individuals may be more inclined to consider the consequences of their disease on the community. In contrast, English-speaking cultures may prioritize individualism and personal autonomy, which could influence their focus on the process of getting disease and the individual experiences. Chinese communication style often emphasizes indirectness and subtlety. When discussing disease, individuals may choose to convey information implicitly, focusing on the consequences and effects rather than explicitly discussing the disease itself. In English-speaking cultures, directness and clarity in communication may be more valued, leading to a greater emphasis on discussing the process of disease. The healthcare systems and practices in different cultures can shape the perception and conceptualization of disease. Chinese traditional medicine, with its holistic approach, emphasizes the consequences of disease and focuses on restoring balance. English-speaking cultures may have healthcare systems that prioritize diagnosis, treatment plans, and the management of the process of getting disease, influencing their perception and conceptualization. The social support systems and stigmas towards the disease can also impact how disease is perceived. Chinese culture places importance on family and community support, which may lead individuals to consider the consequences of their disease on their relationships and social interactions. In English-speaking cultures, there may be more emphasis on the management and coping with disease, potentially reducing the stigma associated with being ill.

　　Historical events and linguistic developments can shape cultural attitudes towards illness or disease. China has a long history of traditional medicine and philosophical influences that prioritize holistic well-being. English-speaking cultures may have been influenced by scientific advancements and a focus on individual health and well-being, which can impact their perception of illness or disease. It's important to note that these are general observations and cultural tendencies, and individuals within each culture may have their own unique perspectives on illness or disease. Nonetheless, considering these socio-cultural factors can help explain the perceptual differences of illness or disease between Chinese and English speakers. During the pandemic, sometimes people in China tend to stigmatize people who are affected by the virus, and blame them for spreading the disease when they travel from place to place. From a socio-cultural perspective, there are several possible reasons that contribute to the perceptual differences of illness or disease between Chinese and English speakers. These reasons include the result-oriented conceptualization of illness in Chinese culture, which focuses on the consequences and outcomes, can contribute to the inclination to stigmatize individuals who are affected by the virus during the pandemic.

When illness or disease is perceived as a result-oriented concept, there is a tendency to attribute blame and responsibility to individuals who are affected. In the case of the pandemic, if someone is seen as responsible for spreading the disease, he or she may be stigmatized and blamed for the negative consequences that follow. Chinese culture places a strong emphasis on the well-being of the common community. Stigmatizing individuals who are affected by the virus can be seen by some as a means of protecting the collective and preventing the spread of the disease. By attributing blame to those individuals, there is a perception that the community's well-being is prioritized over individual circumstances. During a pandemic, there is often fear and uncertainty surrounding the spread of the disease. Result-oriented conceptualization of illness may intensify these emotions, as the focus is on the negative outcomes and consequences. This fear and uncertainty can lead to the stigmatization of individuals who are affected, as a way to distance oneself from the perceived risks and protect one's own well-being.

It's important to acknowledge that stigmatization during a pandemic is a complex phenomenon influenced by various factors, including fear, misinformation, and societal dynamics. While the result-oriented conceptualization of illness or disease in Chinese culture may contribute to the inclination towards stigmatization, it is not the sole determining factor, the individual attitudes and beliefs also play a significant role.

During the pandemic, people from the Western countries are reluctant to wear masks and are unhappy with lockdown measures taken by the government. It seems that Westerners are less tolerant with the strict government policies in preventing the virus from spreading. After the comparison of the conceptualization of illness or disease between English and Chinese from a cognitive linguistic perspective, this book argues that the process-oriented perception of illness in English, of which time is the dominant domain in conceptualization, has an important influence on people's response to measures in curbing the pandemic. Because they are more focused on the time-being and the process, they are less tolerant with emergent measures that limit their freedom, even though the measures are necessary in protecting more people's lives.

The argument that the process-oriented perception of illness or disease in English, influenced by the dominant domain of time in conceptualization, can impact people's response to pandemic measures, specifically their reluctance to wear masks and comply with lockdown measures, can be supported by evidence and explanations from various perspectives. English language and culture exhibit a strong temporal orientation, emphasizing the present moment and immediate outcomes. This temporal focus can lead individuals to prioritize their immediate personal freedoms and well-being over long-term consequences, such as the potential spread of the virus.

English speakers tend to have a future-oriented mindset, valuing progress, individual autonomy, and personal goals. This forward-looking perspective may result in a decreased tolerance for measures that restrict their freedom or disrupt their future plans, even if those measures are necessary for public health. Western cultures, including those influenced by English, often prioritize individualism, emphasizing personal rights, autonomy, and self-expression. This individualistic mindset can lead to a higher degree of resistance to measures that are perceived as infringing upon personal freedoms, as individuals may place a stronger emphasis on their own rights and choices. When individuals perceive their freedom to be threatened or restricted, it can trigger resistance and defiance. In the context of pandemic measures, English speakers may exhibit higher levels of resistance and defiance due to their process-oriented perception of disease, which places a greater emphasis on personal agency and freedom of action.

Western societies, influenced by principles of liberalism and individual rights, often have a tradition of limited government intervention. This cultural backdrop can foster skepticism and resistance towards strict government policies, including pandemic measures, which may be perceived as overly intrusive or paternalistic. The perception of government competence and public trust in institutions can also influence people's willingness to comply with measures. In some Western countries, the historical factors, political polarization, and the skepticism towards authorities may erode trust and contribute to the resistance or non-compliance with pandemic measures.

It's important to note that these perspectives offer insights into possible influences but should not be generalized to all individuals or cultures. Responses to pandemic measures are multifaceted and vary among individuals within a cultural group. Cultural factors interact with individual beliefs, values, and experiences, resulting in diverse responses. Additionally, other factors such as media influence, public health communication strategies, and economic considerations can also contribute to people's attitudes and behaviors during the pandemic.

References

Allwood, J. Semantics as meaning determination with semantic-epistemic operations [J]. *Cognitive Semantics*, 1999 (3): 1 – 17.

Allwood, J. *Cognitive Semantics: Meaning and Cognition* [M]. Amsterdam: John Benjamins Publishing Co., 1999(b).

Barcelona, A. *Metaphor and Metonymy at the Crossroads* [M]. Berlin: De Gruyter Mouton, 2000.

Blank, A. Why do new meanings occur? A cognitive typology of the motivations for lexical semantic change [J]. *Cognitive Linguistics Research*, 1999, 61: 1 – 16.

Brown, P. & Levinson, S. C. *Politeness: Some Universals in Language Usage* [M]. Cambridge: Cambridge University Press, 1987.

Cai, Jun & Zhang, Qingwen. A syntactic-semantic study of implicit eventive causative sentences in Chinese [J]. *Modern Foreign Languages*, 2017, 40 (3): 10.

Cao, Xueqin. *A Dream of Red Mansions* (four volumes) [M]. Translated by Yang Hsien-yi and Gladys Yang. Beijing: Foreign Language Press, 2001.

Cao, Xueqin. *A Dream of Eed Mansions* (two volumes) [M]. Translated by Yang Hsien-yi and Gladys Yang. Beijing: People's Literature Publishing House, 2013.

Cao, Xueqin. *The Story of the Stone* [M]. Translated by David Hawkes. London: Penguin Books, 1973.

Chen, Jiaying. *Philosophy of Language* [M]. Beijing: Peking University Press, 2003.

Chen, Jiaying. Philosophical views of Wittgenstein [J]. *Modern Philosophy*, 2006 (5): 13.

Chen, Junfang. A cognitive contrastive analysis of typical causative motion constructions in English and Chinese under the single-layer constructional grammar framework [J]. *Journal of Xi'an International Studies University*, 2009 (1): 3.

Chen, Ping. On the triadic structure of modern Chinese temporal system [J]. *Chinese Language*, 1988 (6): 401 – 402.

Chomsky, N. *Topics in the Theory of Generative Grammar* [M]. Berlin: De Gruyter Mouton, 1978.

Chu, Ruili & Zhang, Jingyu. A study on the mechanism of metaphorical transformation of the "吃 + NP" construction [J]. *Foreign Languages and Foreign Language Teaching*, 2020 (2): 107 – 115.

Comrie, B. *Language Universals and Linguistic Typology: Syntax and Morphology* [M]. Chicago: The University of Chicago Press, 1989.

Coulson, S. *Semantic Leaps: Frame-Shifting and Conceptual Blending in Meaning Construction* [M]. Cambridge: Cambridge University Press, 2001.

Croft, W. *Syntactic Categories and Grammatical Relations: The Cognitive Organization of Information* [M]. Chicago: The University of Chicago Press, 1991.

Cruse, D A. *Meaning in Language: An Introduction to Semantics and Pragmatics* [M]. Oxford: Oxford University Press, 2004.

Cui, Liang & Wang, Wenbin. Different conceptualizations of actions and time between Chinese and English: Manifestations of temporal-spatial differences [J]. *Theory and Practice in Language Studies*, 2019 (1): 30 – 38.

Dai, Haoyi & Ye, Feisheng. A discussion on Chinese functional grammar based on cognition [J]. *Foreign Linguistics*, 1990 (4): 21 – 27.

Davison, J. *Images and Metaphor: An Analysis of Iban Collective Representation* [D]. London: University of London, 1987a.

Davison, J. *Images and Metaphor: An Analysis of Iban Collective Representation* [M]. School of Oriental and African Studies (United Kingdom), University of London, 1987b.

Deng, Qi & Yang, Zhong. A study on the semantic cognition and semantic functions of sensory adjectives in English and Chinese-taking "cold" and 冷 as examples [J]. *Journal of Foreign Languages*, 2014 (1): 47 – 53.

Fauconnier, G. & Turner, M. Conceptual integration networks [J]. *Cognitive Science*, 1998, 22 (2): 133 – 187.

Fillmore, C. J. Frame semantics and the nature of language [J]. *Annals of the New York Academy of Sciences*, 1976, 280 (1): 20 – 32.

Fillmore, C. J. The mechanisms of "construction grammar" [J]. *Annual Meeting of*

References

the Berkeley Linguistics Society, 1988 (14): 35 –55.

Gawron, J. M. Situations and prepositions [J]. *Linguistics and Philosophy*, 1986 (9): 327 –382.

Gibbs, Jr R. W., Gibbs, R. W. & Gibbs, J. *The Poetics of Mind: Figurative Thought, Language, and Understanding* [M]. Cambridge: Cambridge University Press, 1994.

Goddard, C. & Wierzbicka, A. *Words and Meanings: Lexical Semantics Across Domains, Languages, and Cultures* [M]. Oxford: Oxford University Press, 2013.

Goldberg, A. E. *A Construction Grammar Approach to Argument Structure* [M]. Chicago: The University of Chicago Press, 1995a.

Goldberg, A. E. *Constructions: A Construction Grammar Approach to Argument Structure* [M]. Chicago: The University of Chicago Press, 1995b.

Goldberg, A. E. Constructions: A new theoretical approach to language [J]. *Trends in Cognitive Sciences*, 2003, 7 (5): 219 –224.

Goldberg, A., Brown, K. & Miller, J. Construction grammar [J]. *Cognitive Linguistics Research*, 1996, 34: 401.

Grady, J. *Foundations of Meanings: Primary Metaphors and Primary Scenes* [M]. Berkeley: University of California, 1997.

Hawkes, T. *Structuralism and Semiotics* [M]. London: Methuen, 1977.

Hawks, D. *The Story of Stone* [M]. London: Penguin Books Ltd., 1986.

He, Qingqiang & Wang, Wenbin. Spatial characteristics and personal features of Chinese: Starting from the formation of separable words [J]. *Foreign Languages*, 2016a, 39 (1): 2 –11.

He, Qingqiang & Wang, Wenbin. Temporal and spatial characteristics—A multi-perspective analysis of English-Chinese nominal verb relations [J]. *Modern Foreign Languages*, 2016b, 39 (4): 439 –448.

He, Qingqiang, Wang, Wenbin & Lü, Yufang. Characteristics of Chinese narrative sentences and their second language acquisition research: Based on contrastive analysis of Chinese-English discourse structure [J]. *Language Teaching and Research*, 2019 (6): 1 –11.

Hu, Kaibao. *Introduction to Corpus Translation Studies* [M]. Shanghai: Shanghai Jiao Tong University Press, 2011.

Hu, Xuhui. English causative constructions: A study from the perspective of minimalist program and related theoretical issues [J]. *Foreign Language Teaching and Research*, 2014, 46 (4): 13.

Huang, Chenglong. Causative constructions in typological perspective [J]. *Ethnic Languages*, 2014 (5): 19.

Humboldt, W. *On language: The Diversity of Human Language-Structure and Its Influence on the Mental Development of Mankind* [M]. Cambridge: Cambridge University Press, 1999.

Jackendoff, R. S. *Semantics and Cognition* [M]. Cambridge: The MIT Press, 1985.

Jackendoff, R. S. *Foundations of Language: Brain, Meaning, Grammar, Evolution* [M]. Oxford: Oxford University Press, 2002.

Ji, Y., Hendriks, H. & Hickmann, M. The expression of caused motion events in Chinese and in English: Some typological issues [J]. *Linguistics*, 2011, 49: 1041 – 1077.

Jiang, Shaoyu. Semantic and syntactic changes [J]. *Journal of Soochow University: (Philosophy and Social Sciences Edition)*, 2013 (1): 13.

Kant, I. *Modern Classical Philosophers* [M]. Cambridge: Houghton Mifflin, 1908.

Koffka, K. *Principles of Gestalt Psychology* [M]. London: Routledge, 2013.

Kovecses, Z. *Metaphor in Culture: Universality and Variation* [M]. Cambridge: Cambridge University Press, 2005.

Lakoff, G. Metaphor and war: The metaphor system used to justify war in the Gulf [J]. *Thirty Years of Linguistic Evolution*, 1992 (5): 463 – 481.

Lakoff, G. Cognitive models and prototype theory [J]. *The Cognitive Linguistics Reader*, 2007 (1): 30 – 67.

Lakoff, G. *Women, Fire, and Dangerous Things: What Categories Reveal About the Mind* [M]. Chicago: The University of Chicago Press, 2008.

Lakoff, G. & Johnson, M. *Philosophy in the Flesh: The Embodied Mind and Its Challenge to Western Thought* [M]. New York: Basic Books, 1999.

Lakoff, G. & Johnson, M. *Metaphors We Live By* [M]. Chicago: The University of Chicago Press, 1980/2008.

Langacker, R. W. *Foundations of Cognitive Grammar: Theoretical Prerequisites* (Vol. 1) [M]. Redwood: Stanford University Press, 1987.

Langacker, R. W. *Foundations of Cognitive Grammar* (Vol. 2) [M]. Stanford, CA: Stanford University Press, 1991.

References

Langacker, R. W. *Essentials of Cognitive Grammar* [M]. Oxford: Oxford University Press, 2013.

Levinson, S. C. *Pragmatics* [M]. Cambridge: Cambridge University Press, 1983.

Li, Ying & Xu, Wen. Cognitive study on "head": Metaphor, metonymy, and polysemy [J]. *Foreign Language Teaching*, 2006, 27 (3): 1 – 5.

Liang, Maochen, Li, Wenzhong & Xu, Jiajin. *Tutorial on Corpus Application* [M]. Beijing: Foreign Language Teaching and Research Press, 2010.

Lin, Zhengjun & Yang, Zhong. Diachronic and cognitive analysis of polysemy phenomenon [J]. *Foreign Language Teaching and Research*, 2005 (5): 362 – 367.

Littlemore, J. *Metonymy* [M]. Cambridge: Cambridge University Press, 2015.

Liu, Geng & Wang, Wenbin. English-Chinese temporal-spatial differences from the perspective of word formation [J]. *Journal of Foreign Languages*, 2021 (1): 108 – 115.

Liu, Xiaolin & Wang, Wenbin. On the syntactic and typological effects of quantitative components of Chinese verbs—A contrastive study with English verb systems [J]. *Modern Foreign Languages*, 2009, 32 (1): 42 – 50 + 109.

Liu, Zhengguang & Li, Yi. Comparative study on the temporal and spatial meaning in the use of quantifiers in English and Chinese [J]. *Modern Foreign Languages*, 2020 (2): 147 – 160.

Liu, Zhengguang & Xu, Haoqi. Differences in the conceptualization of time and space between English and Chinese: Temporal-spatial discrete and temporal-spatial homomorphic [J]. *Foreign Language Teaching and Research*, 2019 (2): 163 – 175.

Liu, Zhengguang, Yan, Kefei & Lü, Yingyan. Explanation of the temporal conceptualization differences between English and Chinese in the "before" and "after" temporal opposition [J]. *Modern Foreign Languages*, 2018 (5): 608 – 620.

Liu, Zequan & Yan, Jimiao. A corpus-based study on translator style and translation strategies—Taking reporting verbs in *Dream of the Red Chamber* and their English translations as an example [J]. *Journal of PLA University of Foreign Languages*, 2010 (4): 6.

Lu, Weizhong. A cognitive study on the contrastive meanings of English and Chinese words—On the idea of contrastive cognitive semantics [J]. *Foreign Languages*, 2015 (3): 33 -40.

Luo, Rong & Zhang, Jianli. Interlingual contrastive study of English and Chinese causative constructions [J]. *Journal of Xi'an International Studies University*, 2021, 29 (4): 6.

Luo, Tianhua. Is Chinese an agentive language? —What is and what is not an agentive pattern [J]. *Contemporary Linguistics*, 2021 (1): 16.

Lü, Shuxiang. *Eight Hundred Words in Modern Chinese* [M]. Beijing: The Commercial Press, 1980.

Marlene, Johansson Falck & Lacey, Okonski. Procedure for identifying metaphorical scenes (PIMS): The case of spatial and abstract relations [J]. *Metaphor and Symbol*, 2023, 38 (1): 1 -22.

Martin, Döring & Brigitte, Nerlich. Framing the 2020 coronavirus pandemic: Metaphors, images and symbols [J]. *Metaphor and Symbol*, 2020, 37 (2): 71 -75.

Mehra, A., Kilduff, M. & Brass, D. J. The social networks of high and low self-monitors: Implications for workplace performance [J]. *Administrative Science Quarterly*, 2001, 46 (1): 121 -146.

Ou, Yamei & Liu, Zhengguang. The associative patterns of temporality and grammatical marking in English and Chinese [J]. *Foreign Language Teaching and Research*, 2021, 53 (1): 16 -28 +159.

Pan, Yanyan & Zhang, Hui. A cognitive contrastive study of causative motion constructions in English and Chinese [J]. *Foreign Languages*, 2005 (3): 5.

Payne, T. E. & Payne, T. E. *Describing Morphosyntax: A Guide for Field Linguists* [M]. Cambridge: Cambridge University Press, 1997.

Pederson, E. Geographic and manipulable space in two Tamil linguistic systems [A]. *European Conference on Spatial Information Theory* [C]. Berlin: Springer, 1993: 294 -311.

Peirsman, Yves & Geeraerts, Dirk. Metonymy as a prototypical category [J]. *Cognitive Linguistics*, 2006, 17 (3): 269 -316.

Pustejovsky, J. The syntax of event structure [J]. *Cognition*, 1991(3): 47 -81.

Pustejovsky, J. Type coercion and lexical selection [J]. *Semantics and the Lexicon*, 1993: 73 -94.

References

Pustejovsky, J. & Bouillon, P. Aspectual coercion and logical polysemy [J]. *Journal of Semantics*, 1995, 12 (2): 133 – 162.

Rayson, P. *Matrix: A Statistical Method and Software Tool for Linguistic Analysis through Corpus Comparison* [D]. Lancaster: Lancaster University, 2003.

Rayson, P. From key words to key semantic domains [J]. *International Journal of Corpus Linguistics*, 2008 (3): 519 – 549.

Ren, Shaozeng. Conceptual metaphor and discourse coherence [J]. *Foreign Language Teaching and Research*, 2006, 38 (2): 10.

Ruan, Yongmei & Wang, Wenbin. Grammaticalization differences and temporal-spatial traits of Chinese aspect markers [J]. *Journal of PLA University of Foreign Languages*, 2015, 38 (1): 75 – 82 + 161.

Rubin, N. Figure and ground in the brain [J]. *Nature Neuroscience*, 2001, 4 (9): 857 – 858.

Ruiz, de Mendoza Ibáñez, Francisco, J. & Regina, M. Usón. Levels of description and constraining factors in meaning construction: An introduction to the lexical constructional model [J]. *Construal*, 2008 (3): 355 – 400.

Sartre, J. P. *Being and Nothingness: An Essay in Phenomenological Ontology* [M]. New York: Citadel Press, 2001.

Saussure, F. D., et al. *Course in General Linguistics* [M]. London: Peter Owen, 1959.

Semino, E. *Metaphor in Discourse* [M]. Cambridge: Cambridge University Press, 2008.

Semino, E. Descriptions of pain, metaphor, and embodied simulation [J]. *Metaphor and Symbol*, 2010, 25 (4): 205 – 226.

Semino, E. Corpus linguistics and metaphor [J]. *The Cambridge Handbook of Cognitive Linguistics*, 2017 (4): 463.

Semino, E. "Not soldiers but fire-fighters"—metaphors and Covid-19 [J]. *Health Communication*, 2021, 36 (1): 50 – 58.

Semino, E., Demjén, Z. & Demmen, J. An integrated approach to metaphor and framing in cognition, discourse, and practice, with an application to metaphors for cancer [J]. *Applied Linguistics*, 2018, 39 (5): 625 – 645.

Shao, Bin & He, Lianzhen. A corpus-based study on the cognitive semantics of new words—Taking "Carbon-Cluster Compounds" as an example [J]. *Foreign Language Teaching and Research*, 2012 (4): 7.

Shibatani, M. & Pardeshi, P. The causative continuum [J]. *The Grammar of Causation and Interpersonal Manipulation*, 2002, 48: 85.

Shibatani, M. & Pardeshi, P. The causative continuum [A]. In M. Shibatani (ed.), *The Grammar of Causation and Interpersonal Manipulation* [C]. Amsterdam/Philadelphia: John Benjamins, 2002: 48, 85.

Shu, Dingfang. *Cognitive Semantics* [M]. Shanghai: Shanghai Foreign Language Education Press, 2008.

Shu, Dingfang. *Research on Metaphor and Metonymy* [M]. Shanghai: Shanghai Foreign Language Education Press, 2011.

Song, J. J. *Toward a Typology of Causative Constructions* (Vol. 9) [M]. München: Lincom Europa, 2001.

Sontag, S. *Illness as Metaphor* [M]. New York: Farrar, Straus and Giroux, 1978.

Sun, Chaofen. The boundary and correspondence of Chinese verb system: The aspect marker "le" [J]. *Journal of Teaching Chinese to Speakers of Other Languages Worldwide*, 2022, 36 (1): 19 – 32.

Sweetser, E. *From Etymology to Pragmatics: Metaphorical and Cultural Aspects of Semantic Structure* (Vol. 54) [M]. Cambridge: Cambridge University Press, 1990.

Sybesma, R. *The Mandarin VP* [M]. Amsterdam: Kluwer, 1999.

Talmy, L. *Toward a Cognitive Semantics* [M]. Cambridge: The MIT Press, 2000.

Taylor, J. R. Prepositions: Patterns of polysemization and strategies of disambiguation [A]. In Cornelia Zelinsky-Wibbect (ed.), *The Semantics of Prepositions: From Mental Processing to Natural Language Processing* [C]. Berlin: De Gruyter, 1993: 151 – 175.

Taylor, J. R. *Possessives in English: An Exploration in Cognitive Grammar* [M]. Oxford: Oxford University Press, 1996.

Taylor, J. R. *Linguistic Categorization* [M]. Oxford: Oxford University Press, 2003.

Tian, Hailong. A critical perspective on discourse analysis: From critical linguistics to critical discourse analysis [J]. *Shandong Foreign Language Teaching*, 2006 (2): 8.

Tian, Hailong. *Critical Discourse Analysis: Interpretation, Reflection, Application* [M]. Tianjin: Nankai University Press, 2014.

Ullmann, S. *Semantics: An Introduction to the Science of Meaning* [M]. Oxford:

References

Basil Blackwell, 1962.

Wang, Dongxue & Wang, Wenbin. A comparative study of temporal and spatial perspectives in sentence representation in Chinese, English, and Russian [J]. *Foreign Language Research*, 2018, 35 (4): 8 – 12.

Wang, Shaohua. A cognitive perspective on the metaphorical reasoning mechanism [J]. *Foreign Languages and Foreign Language Teaching*, 2000 (10): 14 – 17.

Wang, Shaohua. The explanatory power of the composite space theory for metaphors [J]. *Foreign Languages*, 2001 (3): 37 – 43.

Wang, Shaohua. Localization of Lakoff's framework theory and the establishment of China's discourse framework system [J]. *The Journal of Chinese Language Studies*, 2022, 19 (1): 30 – 36.

Wang, Wenbin. On the temporal characteristics of English and the spatial characteristics of Chinese [J]. *Foreign Language Teaching and Research*, 2013, 45 (2): 163 – 173.

Wang, Wenbin. Understanding polysemy from the reversibility of form and background—Taking the Chinese verb 吃 and the English verb "make" as examples [J]. *Foreign Languages and Foreign Language Teaching*, 2015 (5): 36 – 41.

Wang, Wenbin & He, Qingqiang. Temporal-spatial differences in Chinese discourse structure—Based on the analysis of anaphoric references in Chinese topic chains and their English translations [J]. *Foreign Language Teaching and Research*, 2016, 48 (5): 657 – 668 + 799.

Wang, Wenbin & Yu, Shanzhi. Spatial and temporal characteristics in Chinese word formation [J]. *Journal of PLA University of Foreign Languages*, 2016, 39 (6): 1 – 8 + 158.

Wang, Wenbin & Zhang, Yuan. Negation representation in English and its temporal-spatial differences in national thinking traits [J]. *Modern Foreign Languages*, 2019, 42 (1): 1 – 12.

Wang, Wenbin & Wu, Juyan. *Lexical Semantics* [M]. Beijing: Foreign Language Teaching and Research Press, 2020.

Wang, Yin. Cognitive translation studies [J]. *Chinese Translators Journal*, 2012, 33 (4): 7.

Wang, Zhanhua. A cognitive investigation of 吃食堂 [J]. *Language Teaching and*

Research, 2000 (2): 58 – 64.

Wu, Ping & Tian, Xingbin. Semantic derivation of causative sentences in Chinese: A case study of 使 sentences and 把 sentences [J]. *Logic Research*, 2018, 11 (1): 14 – 17.

Xin, Bin. Social and cognitive orientation in critical discourse analysis [J]. *Foreign Language Research*, 2007 (6): 6 – 10.

Xin, Bin & Liu, Chen. van Dijk's social-cognitive discourse analysis in brief [J]. *Journal of Foreign Languages*, 2017 (5): 14 – 19.

Xiong, Xueliang. Semantic topology hypothesis of "eat/吃 + NP" expression [J]. *Journal of Tianjin Foreign Studies University*, 2011 (6): 1 – 7.

Xu, Tongqiang. A study on the characteristics of Chinese and the universality of language [J]. *Language Research*, 1999 (4): 1 – 13.

Xu, Shenghuan. The origin, occurrence, and construction of metaphors [J]. *Foreign Language Teaching and Research*, 2014, 46 (3): 11 – 17.

Xun, Endong, et al. Construction of the BCC corpus in the big data context [J]. *Corpus Linguistics*, 2016 (1): 68 – 70.

Yang, Daran. A comparative analysis of causative structures in English: Based on a distributed morphology perspective [J]. *Foreign Language Teaching and Research*, 2021, 53 (2): 163 – 176 + 318.

Yang, Lifang & Wang, Wenbin. A study on the transfer of coherence features of Chinese high school learners—From the perspective of differences in temporality and spatiality in English [J]. *Chinese Foreign Language*, 2017, 14 (1): 68 – 76.

Yuan, Hongmei & Wang, Shaohua. Critical metaphor analysis of news headlines on Covid-19 in mainstream US media involving China [J]. *Journal of Zhejiang International Studies University*, 2022 (5): 9.

Zhang, Bojiang. Functional explanation of word-class usage [J]. *Chinese Language*, 1994 (5): 8.

Zhang, Bojiang. When to use the 把 construction—Based on a textual investigation [J]. *Journal of World Chinese Language Teaching*, 2020, 34 (2): 14.

Zhang, Cun, Lin, Zhengjun & Jin, Shengxi. What else besides war: Deliberate metaphors framing Covid-19 in Chinese online newspaper editorials [J]. *Metaphor and Symbol*, 2022, 37: 2, 114 – 126.

References

Zhang, Hui. *Studies in Cognitive Semantics* [M]. Shanghai: Shanghai Foreign Language Education Press, 2011.

Zhang, Hui & Jiang, Long. On the fusion of cognitive linguistics and critical discourse analysis [J]. *Journal of Foreign Languages*, 2008 (5): 8.

Zhang, Jianli. A comparative network analysis of the polysemy of 心 in English [J]. *Journal of Zhejiang University (Humanities and Social Sciences)*, 2006 (3): 161 – 168.

Zhang, Wangxi. The displacement schema of 把 sentences [J]. *Language Teaching and Research*, 2001 (3): 10.

Zhang, Jidong, Liu, Lian & Liu, Ping. A study on the linguistic features of "causative constructions" based on the contemporary English corpus of the United States—Taking "into V-ing causative constructions" as an example [J]. *Foreign Language Teaching*, 2019, 40 (4): 6.

Zhang, Hui. Critical cognitive linguistics and sociorecontextualization [J]. *Journal of Shenzhen University (Humanities and Social Sciences Edition)*, 2022, 39 (1): 9.

Zhang, Ren. Semantic emergence of word meaning—Use imprint and schema [J]. *Modern Foreign Languages*, 2018 (3): 306 – 319.

Zhang, Wei & Wang, Shaohua. ICM analysis of disease metaphor expression in news publications [J]. *Journal of Nanjing Audit University*, 2011 (4): 5.

Zhang, Wei & Wang, Shaohua. Cognitive analysis of deliberate metaphors in COVID-19 news reports [J]. *Journal of Tianjin Foreign Studies University*, 2020, 27 (2): 15.

Zhao, Chaoyong & Wang, Wenbin. Error analysis of Chinese learners' temporality and spatiality in English acquisition: A perspective of differences in temporality and spatiality between English and Chinese [J]. *Foreign Language Teaching Theory and Practice*, 2017 (4): 13 – 21.

Zhao, Chaoyong & Wang, Wenbin. A study on the teaching effectiveness based on the comparative method of temporality and spatiality—From the perspective of differences in temporality and spatiality in English [J]. *Computer-Assisted Foreign Language Teaching*, 2020 (3): 81 – 87 + 13.

Zhao, Yanfang. *Introduction to Cognitive Linguistics* [M]. Shanghai: Shanghai Foreign Language Education Press, 2001.

Zhou, Ruirui & Li, Jianxue. A study on the grammatical metaphors in causative constructions [J]. *Journal of Mudanjiang University*, 2017, 26 (11): 4.

Zhu, Qingxiang. Qualitative characteristics of the direct object of the 把 sentence from the perspective of interactive information [J]. *Language Sciences*, 2019, 18 (4): 14.

曹雪芹. 红楼梦[M]. 北京:人民文学出版社,2019.

老舍. 我这一辈子[M]. 上海:上海阅文信息技术有限公司,2016.

王永战,吴月. 让每个孩子都闪光(教改一线·校长和学校的故事)[N]. 人民日报,2022-06-19.